LEAN & GREEN DIET

Table of Content

INTRODUCTION

Consumers have long been drawn to the convenience of meal replacement diets that take the guesswork out of weight loss. One popular meal replacement plan is the Optavia Diet. By combining "fuelings" (shakes, bars, and other pre-packaged foods) with a six-small-meals-per-day philosophy, the Optavia Diet aims to help people lose weight by consuming small amounts of calories throughout the day. Optavia adds a social support component by offering access to a health coach who can answer questions and provide encouragement.

To help you decide if the program could help you achieve your weight loss goals, here's a look at how the Optavia Diet works, as well as the plan's pros and cons. The Optavia diet is a meal replacement plan. Followers eat a certain number of 'fuelings' per day (plus one homemade meal) resulting in calorie reduction and weight loss. Experts worry that it's unsustainable; many will regain weight when transitioning off the meal replacements.

The Optavia Diet might sound unfamiliar, as the name itself hasn't been around very long. You're more likely to have heard of the diet by its previous name, Take Shape for Life, which was rebranded as Optavia in July 2017. Take Shape for Life began as a subsidiary of Medifast, a weight-loss product company founded in 1980 by a medical doctor named Dr. William Vitale. When it was introduced in 2002, the intent of Take Shape for Life was to offer Medifast's products in an online format better suited to the digital age. The Optavia Diet is not intended for a specific audience, but it tends to appeal to people who want to stop "overthinking" an eating plan.

With Optavia's popular "5 & 1" plan, five out of the six small meals per day are pre-planned and pre-packaged, eliminating the need for any big decisions when it's time to eat. Optavia tends to be a favorite among people with a busy lifestyle, but the plan's reduced-calorie approach is intended for anyone looking to lose weight. Still, the Optavia Diet has not been without controversy. Critics have called the plan a pyramid scheme because of its multi-level structure, and the sales and promotions aspect of the program can be a turnoff for potential customers.

How to Spot a Weight Loss Scam

Users who complete Optavia's program are encouraged to become coaches, sell the company's products, and recruit new sales representatives.

L ike other meal replacement diets, the Optavia Diet provides users with its own array of branded products that take the place of several meals throughout the day. Optavia offers diet plans for goals of weight loss and weight maintenance.

The "5 & 1" plan is the most popular and is designed for rapid weight loss. On this plan, users eat five of Optavia's "fuelings" and one low-calorie "lean and green" homemade meal per day. Optavia's other plans, the "3 & 3" and "4 & 2 & 1", combine "real" meals with meal replacements. These plans are best-suited to users who want to lose weight slowly or maintain their current weight.

On all of Optavia's plans, both "fuelings" and "lean and green" homemade meals are kept within strict calorie ranges.

The Optavia Diet deviates from health and nutrition guidelines encouraged by the United States Department of Agriculture (USDA) in several areas.

The USDA's Dietary Guidelines for Americans 2015-2020 estimate that a healthy adult requires 1600 to 3000 calories per day, depending on their activity level. Although Optavia's 5 & 1 plan is intended for weight loss, the 800 to 1000 calorie count per day is an extreme reduction from the USDA's recommendation.

One area where Optavia deviates from USDA recommendations is in terms of macronutrients specifically, carbohydrates. Optavia's plans reportedly provide 80 to 100 grams of carbohydrates per day. In other words, about 40% of the diet's daily calories come from carbs, whereas the USDA Dietary Guidelines recommend a diet that is 45 to 65% carbohydrates.

The USDA also emphasizes that a healthy eating plan includes grains and dairy products, which are not represented in Optavia's 5 & 1 plan.

There are several popular diet plans that are similar to Optavia, but with key differences that might influence whether they are a good fit for your goals.

SlimFast Diet

When you think of meal replacements, SlimFast probably comes to mind first. While the food and product aspects of SlimFast and Optavia's plans are similar, there are some key differences.

SlimFast's array of meal replacement products is similar in nutrition but you won't find as much variety as with Optavia's plan. However, an attribute of SlimFast is that it does offer meal replacement lines that comply with special diets, such as keto and diabetic weight loss.

If you like the idea of having built-in social support and coaching, that's a key feature of Optavia's plan that you won't find with a SlimFast diet.

Special K Diet

Another popular meal replacement plan is the Special K diet. To follow the two-week "challenge," you'll replace two meals a day with Special K cereal or another Special K product, then eat your usual dinner.

The Special K diet is essentially a "quick-fix" or "crash diet," and is not intended for longer-term use. Optavia's 5 & 1 plan also offers quick weight loss but with a bit more variety than two meals of cereal a day.

With Optavia, you can also transition to the 3 & 3 or 4 & 2 & 1 plans for weight maintenance once you meet your initial goal.

If cost is your main consideration, two weeks' of the Special K diet is certainly a cheaper option than most diet programs including Optavia's.

Do "Quick Fix" Weight Loss Diets Work?

Like Optavia, Nutrisystem is a meal replacement company that sends users pre-made, pre-packaged foods that take the planning and guesswork out of meal prep and planning. However, in contrast to Optavia's "fuelings," Nutrisystem's products more closely resemble typical meals.

Nutrisystem's food choices, such as pizza, sandwiches, and mac and cheese, are intended to stand in for all three
meals a day. If the social support aspect of diet programs appeals to you, Nutrisystem also offers support services from on-call counselors.

If you thrive on structure and need to lose weight quickly, the Optavia Diet could be a good fit for you. With its extremely low-calorie eating plans, it's certainly likely to help you shed pounds; however, whether that weight loss will stick once you go off the diet is debatable.

Before you begin any meal replacement diet, carefully consider whether you can realistically follow it, decide how much money you can invest, and determine the degree of hunger and interruption to your social routine you are comfortable with. If you decide to opt for Optavia and succeed with your short-term weight loss goals, make sure you become educated about healthy eating so you can keep the weight off long-term. Also, remember that a calorie-restricted commercial diet is not the only way to slim down. Talk to your healthcare provider or a registered dietitian about simple changes you can make to create a more satisfying nutritious meal plan to help you achieve your goals.

I f you're investing the most popular diet plans to lose weight, you'll find the Optimal Weight 5 & 1 plan on your list of programs to consider. But trying to choose the right plan can be tricky and there are many different factors to evaluate.

Dieters on the OPTAVIA 5 & 1 Plan eat five commercially prepared meal replacements each day plus one Lean & Green meal that you prepare yourself. Meal replacements are familiar foods like mashed potatoes, brownies, pasta, muffins, or soups that have been engineered to provide more protein, less carbohydrate, and limited fat.

Taste

Success on the 5 & 1 Plan requires that you eat a lot of OPTAVIA food. There are plenty of options to choose from and I took a week to sample several popular items. The verdict?

While the foods don't necessarily taste like their "real-world" counterparts, the food didn't taste bad.

For example, the brownie was warm and somewhat chocolatey but didn't necessarily offer the satisfaction of a regular brownie. Mashed potatoes were bland but the consistency was good and I found them modestly satisfying. If you don't have time to cook your own Lean & Green meal (a combination of lean protein and non-starchy vegetables) you can rely on an OPTAVIA Flavors of Home meal. The microwavable meals do not need to be refrigerated so they are quick and convenient. Choices include Turkey Meatball Marinara, Chicken with Rice and Vegetables, and Chicken Cacciatore.

So, how do they taste? I only tried one (Chicken Cacciatore) and would suggest that dieters opt to cook their own meal.

Coaching and Support

OPTAVIA offers several tools to help guide you through the weight loss process:

Online tools to record data: You can record your meal plans, weight loss, exercise, and measurements online or with the Mobile App. Dieters can use these tools at home, at work, or on-the-go to keep their diet journals up to date. As you progress or when you hit struggles you can review data to make changes as necessary.

Community support: Through the online community, you can connect with other dieters to share tips, get feedback about struggles, share successes, and make new friends. Many times, it is the support of fellow dieters that means the most when you are trying to lose weight.

Physician support: Some dieters gain access to OPTAVIA foods and programs through their physicians. For clients with health considerations, this may be the safest option. Not all physicians, however, are part of the nationwide network. You may have to go outside of your network to find a physician who is.

Health coaches: OPTAVIA offers clients the option to buy foods through agents they call "health coaches." These are not certified health professionals but rather agents who have demonstrated knowledge of the OPTAVIA program and who earn income from selling and promoting the foods.[4] While some of the coaches may carry outside credentials, clients should not assume that they have expertise in the fields of health, nutrition, diet, or weight loss.

Cost

119 servings of OPTAVIA food will cost $414.60.*

The minimum total cost for a 12-16 week program might range from $1385.40 (12 weeks) to $1878.15 (16 weeks) for the initial part of the plan.

But there are other costs to consider. Of course, you need to factor in the cost of your home-cooked Lean & Green Meal. Alternatively, if you choose to eat OPTAVIA's Flavors of Home meals, add at least $30 per week. Lastly, as you transition off the plan, you'll still eat OPTAVIA meal replacements for at least 6 weeks. This could add several hundred dollars to your bottom line.

Weight Loss

Every dieter is different and different weight loss plans work for different people. Evaluate these pros and cons of Medifast before you make a final decision about whether this is the best diet for you.

- **Pros**

The benefits of this plan include:

Simplicity: You won't have to keep detailed notes or count calories while you lose weight on OPTAVIA. You simply need to count to five. Foods are exceptionally easy to cook and take a few minutes to prepare.

Convenient: There is no excuse not to stick to this diet. The foods are microwavable and some need no preparation at all. You can easily throw a meal replacement packet or a bar into your purse or briefcase for diet-friendly eating on the go. This would be a good diet for people who have very hectic schedules, travel often or don't have time to cook.

- **Cons**

Possible drawbacks of this diet are:

Food taste: While most of the food wasn't bad, it wasn't great either. Foodies and people who love to cook may suffer on this plan. For this reason, some dieters may struggle to stick to the plan long enough to lose their weight.

Potentially difficult transition: The type of foods offered on the plan may make it difficult to transition off the plan when you've reached your goal. OPTAVIA guides clients through a reasonable transition program where they step down and add real-world foods to their diet. But if dieters grab the high-fat and high-carb real-world counterparts to the foods they've gotten used to (like brownies, mashed potatoes or cheese curls), they may gain weight.

Expense: The OPTAVIA 5 & 1 Plan is not cheap. But most plans that offer convenience tend to be pricey. If you choose to go on the program, make sure that you plan for the total cost of your entire weight loss journey so that you don't quit halfway through because you can't afford it.

Take plenty of time to evaluate this or any diet before you invest your money and time. Ask yourself five important questions to make sure you get a program that fits your lifestyle and your needs.

S tudies haven't shown major problems with OPTAVIA. Side effects might include leg cramps, dizziness or fatigue, headaches, loose skin, hair loss, rashes, gas, diarrhea, bad breath, gallstones or gallbladder disease for those at risk, constipation and (for women) menstrual changes.

The apparent absence of noteworthy risks does not mean OPTAVIA is safe for everyone. Pregnant women and those younger than 13 years old shouldn't be on any program, while teens, nursing mothers, people with gout and others should stick to those programs geared toward them (after clearing it with their doctors, of course). Older, sedentary adults and people who exercise more than 45 minutes a day should avoid the 5&1 Program. People with serious illnesses like cancer, liver disease, kidney disease or an eating disorder shouldn't follow any plan unless their health care providers have cleared them as recovered and stabilized.

If you're on any medications especially warfarin, lithium, diabetes medication or medications for high blood pressure talk to your doctor before starting any of the programs, the company advises.

Is Optavia Diet a heart-healthy diet?

OPTAVIA may possibly be heart healthy, but no more than many other diets. OPTAVIA contends its Fuelings are low in fat and cholesterol, and many contain enough high-quality soy protein to meet the Food and Drug Administration's Heart Health claim.

OPTAVIA represents the community of coaches and lifestyle brand launched in 2017. Previous studies were conducted using some products, not the new OPTAVIA products. While the OPTAVIA products represent a new line, Medifast has advised U.S. News that they have an identical macronutrient profile and as such are interchangeable with the Medifast products. Therefore, we believe these studies are relevant when evaluating this diet.

In the 2017 Medifast-sponsored study in the journal Nutrition and Diabetes, participants significantly reduced their blood pressure. A study found that overweight and obese participants following the 4&2&1 Plan significantly improved their blood pressure. In the 2010 Nutrition Journal study described in the weight-loss section, researchers reported declines in blood pressure, pulse rate and blood levels of C-reactive protein, a marker of inflammation that may predict heart disease risk, in the Medifast and control groups at week 40. The study also reported on waist size and amount of abdominal fat, which are thought to be indicators of heart disease risk. At week 40, Medifast dieters had lost an average of about 4 inches around the waist, the control group about 1 1/2 inches. The abdominal "fat rating" for both groups had decreased as well, but the Medifast group performed slightly better. At week 40, total cholesterol was not significantly lower for the Medifast group but had dropped appreciably for the control group. Neither group showed improved levels of triglycerides, a fatty substance that in excess has been linked to heart disease, at 40 weeks.

In the Diabetes Educator study, the Medifast dieters had significantly higher good HDL cholesterol and lower systolic blood pressure after 86 weeks, but neither change was significant when compared to the control group.

Optavia Meal Plan

- **Breakfast Serving Size**

¾ cup ready-to-eat unsweetened cereal

1 cup skim or low-fat milk 1 Starch

1 Dairy

- **Mid-Morning Fueling**

Optimal Health Strawberry Yogurt Bar 1 Optimal Health Fueling

- **Lunch**

½ cup cooked cauliflower

3 oz. grilled chicken ¾ cup low-fat yogurt 1 Vegetable

1 Protein

1 Dairy

- **Mid-Afternoon Fueling**

Optimal Health Strawberry Banana Smoothie 1 Optimal Health Fueling

- **Dinner**

2 cups raw spinach

1 cup total diced tomatoes, cucumbers, and mushrooms

3 oz. baked yellowfin tuna

2 Tbsp low-fat salad dressing

1 small apple

1 Protein

1 Fat

1 Fruit

1.   **GARLIC CHICKEN WITH ZOODLES**

This creamy garlic chicken is one of our favorite lean and green recipes! It's colorful and packed full of flavor without the guilt!

Prep Time: 15 mins

Cook Time: 15 mins

Total Time: 30 mins

INGREDIENTS

1 1/2 lbs boneless skinless chicken breasts

1 T olive oil

1 C low fat plain greek yogurt

1/2 C chicken broth

1/2 tsp garlic powder

1/2 tsp italian seasoning

1/4 C parmesan cheese

1 C spinach, chopped

3-6 slices sun dried tomatoes

1 T chopped garlic

1 1/2 C zucchini cut into thin noodles

INSTRUCTIONS

HOW TO COOK THE CHICKEN

Heat the oil in a large skillet on medium.

Using paper towels, pat the chicken breast dry, sprinkle with salt and pepper for taste and place in hot oil.

Cook on medium high for for 3-5 minutes on each side or until brown on each side and until no longer pink in center.

Remove chicken and set aside on a plate.

Add the yogurt, chicken broth, garlic powder, Italian seasoning, and parmesan cheese into the large skillet.

Whisk over medium high heat until it starts to thicken.

Add the spinach and sun dried tomatoes.

Simmer until the spinach starts to wilt.

Add the chicken back to the pan and serve over zucchini noodles.

HOW TO COOK THE ZOODLES

Preheat oven to 350 degrees F.

Using vegetable spiraler, cut zucchini into the shape of spiral noodles.

Place parchment paper on a large baking sheet. Spread and arrange zoodles and toss with sea salt. Be sure to spread them thin so they don't stick together.

Bake for 15 min for al dente. Add a couple minutes if you want them softer.

Serve right away.

2. **Optavia Biscuit Pizza Ingredients**

1 sachet Optavia Buttermilk Cheddar and Herb Biscuit

2 Tbsp water

1 Tbsp tomato sauce

1 Tbsp low fat shredded cheese

Instructions

Preheat oven or toaster to 350 degrees F.

Stir together biscuit and water and spread into a thin circle on parchment paper and cook for 10 minutes.

Add tomato sauce then shredded cheese and bake for a few more minutes, until the cheese has melted.

3.   **Lean and Green**

Prep: 10 mins

Total: 10 mins

Servings: 1

Ingredient

1 cup fresh spinach

1 banana

½ green apple
4 hulled strawberries

4 (1 inch) pieces frozen mango

⅓ Cup whole milk

1 scoop vanilla protein powder (Optional)

1 teaspoon honey

Directions

Blend spinach, banana, apple, strawberries, mango, milk, protein powder, and honey together in a blender until smooth.

4.   **Medifast Chicken Stir Fry**

Minutes to Prepare: 10

Minutes to Cook: 10

Number of Servings: 2

Ingredients

12 oz skinless, boneless chicken breast

1 cup chopped red bell pepper

1 cup chopped green bell pepper

8 oz (1 cup) broccoli slaw

1/2 cup chicken broth

2 tbs low sodium no carb soy sauce

1 tsp crushed red pepper

Directions

Sautee peppers and broccoli slaw in chicken broth. Add soy sauce, add chicken and red pepper. Cook for a few more minutes until peppers are tender.

5. **OPTAVIA Mini Mac In A Bowl**

INGREDIENTS

2 Tablespoons yellow or white onion; diced
5 ounces 95-97% Lean Ground Beef

2 Tablespoons Wish-Bone Light Thousand Island dressing

1/8 teaspoon White Vinegar

1/8 teaspoon Onion Powder

3 cups Romaine Lettuce; shredded

2 Tablespooons Reduced-Fat Cheddar Cheese; shredded

1 ounce Dill Pickle Slices

1 teaspoon sesame seeds

Cooking Spray

INSTRUCTIONS

1. Heat a small, lightly greased skillet over medium-high heat. Add the onion & cook until fragrant, about 2-3 minutes. Add the beef and cook until fully browned.

2. Meanwhile, mix together the dressing, vinegar and onion powder.

3. To assemble: Top lettuce with the ground beef and sprinkle with cheese. Top with pickle slices. Drizzle with sauce, and sprinkle with sesame seeds.

6.   **Avocado Citrus Shrimp Salad**

YIELDS 2 Servings

PREP TIME: 25 mins

COOK TIME: 5 mins

TOTAL TIME: 30 mins

INGREDIENTS

½   lb wild caught shrimp (uncooked)

1 avocado

1 head green leaf lettuce (or any other mild lettuce)

2 tbsp olive oil (try The Crescent Olive's Lime Extra Virgin Olive Oil!)

Sea salt, pepper, cayenne, cumin, garlic powder, onion powder

Juice of lemon or lime

Microgreens (optional)

DIRECTION

Prepare the lettuce:

Wash, dry, and chop lettuce. Arrange on 2 plates and set aside.

Prepare the Shrimp:

Remove tails from shrimp and place in strainer to remove excess liquid.

Transfer to mixing bowl and combine with spices. Toss gently to coat evenly.

Heat 1 tbsp. olive oil in a skillet over medium-low heat.

Cook shrimp for 2-3 minutes on one side, flip and cook for 1-2 minutes on the second side. Cover, turn off heat, and let shrimp continue to cook through for a few more minutes.

Prepare the Avocado:

Slice avocado in half around the pit. On each side, score the flesh to create cubes of avocado. Invert skin to release avocado cubes. Place on top of lettuce.

Prepare the Dressing:

In a small bowl, combine 2 tbsp. olive oil, juice of 1/2 lemon or lime, salt and pepper. Whisk together until combined.

Put it all together:

Arrange cooked shrimp on top of lettuce.

Using a spoon, distribute dressing over salads.

Top with more of the spices that were used to season the shrimp.

Top with microgreens (if using) and serve immediately!

The olive oil and lemon juice help your body to assimilate and absorb the fat soluble nutrients in the green lettuce, the citrus prevents the avocado from browning, and all ingredients compliment each other for a complete meal!

7.   BROCCOLI TACO BOWL

This Broccoli Taco Bowl is Gluten Free and helps you stay on track with your weight loss goals!

PREP TIME: 2 mins

COOK TIME: 10 mins

TOTAL TIME: 12 mins

SERVINGS 1

INGREDIENTS

4- oz lean ground hamburger

1- oz shredded cheddar cheese

1 1/4 cup broccoli, cut into bite sized pieces

1/4 cup Rotel tomatoes

1/4 teaspoon garlic powder

1/4 teaspoon onion powder

1/4 teaspoon salt, divided

Pinch of red pepper flakes

2 tablespoons low sodium chicken stock

DIRECTIONS

Put your broccoli in a bowl with your chicken stock and cover with plastic wrap. Put in the microwave for 4 minutes, or until tender and cooked.

In a large skillet brown your hamburger and drain the grease if needed when it's done.

Add your Rotel tomatoes, garlic powder, onion powder, salt, and red pepper flakes and stir well.

When your broccoli is finished cooking then add it to your skillet and toss with the hamburger mixture.
Add everything to a bowl and top with your shredded cheddar cheese.

8.   Mac & Cheese: The Lean Green

COOK TIME: 30 minutes

Ingredients

1 lb small shell pasta (455 g)

3 ½ cups whole milk (840 mL)

8 tablespoons unsalted butter

2 cups shredded american cheese (200 g)

2 teaspoons kosher salt

½ teaspoon ground black pepper

2 cups broccoli floret (300 g), steamed

½ cup shredded parmesan cheese (55 g)

Preparation

In a large pot over medium heat, combine the pasta and milk. Bring the milk to a simmer and cook until the pasta is tender, 8–10 minutes.

Once the pasta is cooked, remove the pan from the heat and add the butter, American cheese, salt, and pepper.
Stir until fully combined. Fold in the broccoli.

Divide between serving bowls and top with the Parmesan cheese.

Enjoy!

9.   OPTAVIA CLOUD BREAD

Yields: 3 Servings

INGREDIENTS

1/16 teaspoon Cream of Tartar

3 Eggs

1/2 cup Fat-Free 0% Plain Greek Yogurt

1 packet sweetener

DIRECTION

At least 1/2 hour before making, put the whisk attachment and Kitchen Aid Bowl in the freezer.

Preheat oven to 300 degrees. Get the bowl & whisk attachment out of the Freezer. Separate the eggs.

Put the whites in the Kitchen Aid Bowl and the yolks in a different medium-sized bowl. In the medium-sized bowl with the yolks, mix in the Greek Yogurt and sweetener. In the bowl with the egg whites, add in the cream of tartar.

Beat this mixture until the egg whites form stiff peaks. Take the egg yolk mixture and gently fold it into the egg whites.

Do not over-stir.

Put parchment paper on a baking tray.

Spray with cooking spray.

Scoop out 6 equally-sized "blobs" of the "dough" onto the parchment paper. Bake 25-35 minutes (check at 25 minutes.

In some ovens, they are done at this point).

They will get brownish on the top and crackled. Most people prefer them cold vs warm. Many people like to re-heat in a toaster or toast oven to get them somewhat crispy.

10.   **Optavia Pizza Hack**

Prep Time: 10 mins

Cook Time: 16 mins

Servings: 1

Equipment

Parchment Paper

2 Baking sheets

Saute pan

Ingredients

Pizza Crust

1 packet Garlic Smashed Potato Packet 1 Fueling

2 Egg Whites* 1/7 Leanest

1 tsp Baking Powder** 2 Condiments

Pizza Toppings

1/4 cup Pizza Sauce*** 1 Green

1/2 cup Sliced white mushrooms 1 Green

3 oz Reduced Fat Shredded Mozzarella 3/4 Lean

1.5 oz Ground Beef 1/4 Leaner

2 Black Olives sliced 1/4 Fat

Instructions

Bake Crust

Preheat Oven to 400 degrees.

Mix together the garlic potato packet and baking powder.

Add egg whites and stir until combined.

Pour batter onto parchment paper lined baking sheet.

Top with another piece of parchment paper and spread out the batter to a 1/8 of an inch circle.

Top with second baking sheet so the crust is sandwiched between the two sheets.
Bake for 8 minutes or until crust is golden brown.

Add Toppings to Pizza

While crust is baking, brown ground beef in a saute pan, wash the mushrooms, and measure your toppings.

When crust is done, pull out of oven put aside top baking sheet and peel back the top layer of parchment paper.

Be careful as paper might stick at this step.

Layer pizza sauce, shredded cheese, and toppings.

Bake for another 8 minutes. When the pizza is ready it should slide right off the parchment paper and easily transfer to a plate.

11.   **Chicken Pesto Pasta**

This lightened up Lean Green Chicken Pesto Pasta tastes like spring in a bite. A quick low-fat pesto, tossed with chickpea pasta, chicken, and fresh mozzarella, you will get yourself a flavorful and nutritious meal in under 30 minutes!

Makes: 5 servings (just over 8 cups)

Prep Time: 15 minutes

Total Time: 30 minutes

Ingredients

Kale Pesto

3 cups (48g) raw kale (stems removed)

2 cup (12g) fresh basil

2 tablespoons (28g) olive oil

3 tablespoons lemon juice

3 garlic cloves

¼   teaspoon salt

Pasta Salad

2 cups (280g) cooked chicken breast (diced)

6 oz (176g) uncooked "Barilla" rotini chickpea pasta

1 cup (20g) arugula or baby spinach

3oz (84g) "Bel Gioioso" fresh mozzarella (diced)

Optional: additional basil leaves or red pepper flakes for garnish
Instructions

Make the pesto by adding the kale, basil, olive oil, garlic cloves, lemon juice, and salt to a food processor. Blend until smooth. Season to taste with additional salt and pepper.

Cook pasta according to package directions. Strain, reserving ¼ cup cooking liquid. In a large bowl, mix together the cooked pasta, diced chicken, pesto, arugula or spinach, reserved pasta liquid, and mozzarella and toss until combined. Sprinkle with extra chopped basil or red pepper flakes (if desired).

Serve chilled or warm. This pasta salad is delicious on its own, as a salad mix-in, or as a side! Store leftovers in an airtight container in the refrigerator for 3-5 days. Enjoy!

12. **Crockpot Chili**

This lean and Green Crock Pot Chili Recipe is a yummy lightened up Green Chili recipe made in the slow cooker and is only 241 calories per serving!

Prep Time: 10 minutes

Cook Time: 5 hours

Total Time: 5 hours 10 minutes

Ingredients

1 pound boneless skinless chicken breasts cut into 3/4 inch pieces

1/2 cup chopped onions

2 tsp Ground Cumin

1 to 2 tsp garlic

1/2 tsp chili powder

Salt and pepper (about 1/4 tsp each)

2 cans of fat free chicken broth

1 can of green enchilada sauce (or 1 1/2 cup of salsa verde)

8 6-inch corn tortillas broken into very small pieces (divided)

3/4 cup of corn

2 cans of beans, drained and rinsed (Black or pinto)

1 tsp cornstarch

1/2 evaporated milk or (1/3 cup of dry milk and 1/2 cup water)

Optional toppings:

2 tsp snipped fresh cilantro

Sour cream

Shredded Cheese

Instructions

Add chicken, chopped onion, chicken broth, enchilada sauce, spices and half of the broken up corn tortillas to the crock-pot and mix everything together.

Cook on low for 4 hours.

Once the chili has cooked for 4 hours, add the corn, beans, and the rest of the broken up tortillas to the crock pot.

Stir the cornstarch into the evaporated milk (or dry milk/water) until completely dissolved.

Mix cornstarch Mixture into the chili.

Cook on low for 1 more hour.

Serve and then top with optional sour cream, shredded cheese and cilantro.

Enjoy!

13. **Green Beans, Ground Turkey and Rice**

This ground turkey and rice recipe gets a major upgrade by adding crispy green beans and a bit of sesame oil for some extra flavor.

Prep Time: 15 minutes

Cook Time: 13 minutes

Total Time: 28 minutes

4 Servings

Ingredients

1 Tbsp. + 1 tsp. sesame oil

1 lb. 93% lean ground turkey raw

5 cups green beans ends trimmed

Sea salt (or Himalayan salt) and

ground black pepper to taste;

optional 1⅓ cups brown rice

cooked

Instructions

Heat oil in large skillet over medium-high heat.

Add turkey; cook, stirring frequently, for 4 to 6 minutes, or until browned and no longer pink.

Add green beans; cook, covered, stirring occasionally, for 4 to 6 minutes, or until green beans are tender crisp.

Season with salt and pepper (if desired); mix well.

Serve each portion over ⅓ cup rice.

14.   LEAN AND GREEN GARLIC CHICKEN WITH ZOODLES

This creamy garlic chicken is one of our favorite lean and green recipes! It's colorful and packed full of flavor without the guilt!

Prep Time: 15 mins

Cook Time: 15 mins

Total Time: 30 mins

INGREDIENTS

1 1/2 lbs boneless skinless chicken breasts

1 T olive oil

1 C low fat plain greek yogurt

1/2 C chicken broth

1/2 tsp garlic powder

1/2 tsp italian seasoning

1/4 C parmesan cheese

1 C spinach, chopped

3-6 slices sun dried tomatoes

1 T chopped garlic

1 1/2 C zucchini cut into thin noodles

INSTRUCTIONS

HOW TO COOK THE CHICKEN

Heat the oil in a large skillet on medium.

Using paper towels, pat the chicken breast dry, sprinkle with salt and pepper for taste and place in hot oil.

Cook on medium high for 3-5 minutes on each side or until brown on each side and until no longer pink in center.

Remove chicken and set aside on a plate.

Add the yogurt, chicken broth, garlic powder, Italian seasoning, and parmesan cheese into the large skillet.

Whisk over medium high heat until it starts to thicken.

Add the spinach and sun dried tomatoes.

Simmer until the spinach starts to wilt.

Add the chicken back to the pan and serve over zucchini noodles.

HOW TO COOK THE ZOODLES

Preheat oven to 350 degrees F.

Using vegetable spiraler, cut zucchini into the shape of spiral noodles.

Place parchment paper on a large baking sheet. Spread and arrange zoodles and toss with sea salt. Be sure to spread them thin so they don't stick together.

Bake for 15 min for al dente. Add a couple minutes if you want them softer.

Serve right away.

15.   BBQ Turkey Burgers

Fire up the grill for BBQ Turkey Burgers tonight! BBQ Turkey Burgers are ultra-moist and tasty, making them a great alternative to traditional high-fat beef patties. Sweet onion is a tasty contradiction to tangy BBQ sauce. Try it with grilled pineapple too.

Yield: Makes 4 burgers (serving size: 1 bbq turkey burger)

Ingredients

1 pound ground dark-meat turkey

1 garlic clove, minced

1/2 teaspoon paprika

1/4 teaspoon ground cumin

Pinch of kosher salt

1/4 teaspoon freshly ground black pepper

4 slices sweet onion, grilled

1/4 cup barbecue sauce

4 (1.6-oz) sesame seed buns, toasted

Directions

In medium bowl, gently mix together turkey, garlic, paprika, and cumin.

Form turkey into 4 (4-inch) patties; season with salt and pepper.

Heat grill to medium-high; cook, turning once, until burgers are just cooked through (about 7 minutes per side).
Serve with desired toppings and buns.

16.   **Energy-Revving Quinoa**

This meatless meal of Energy-Revving Quinoa keeps you

energized between meals or after a workout. Yield: Makes 1

serving (serving size: 1 1/2 cups)

Ingredients

1 cup cooked quinoa

1/3 cup canned low-sodium black beans, drained and rinsed

1 small tomato, chopped

1 scallion, sliced

1 teaspoon olive oil

1 teaspoon fresh lemon juice

Pinch of salt

Pinch of freshly ground black pepper

Directions

In a medium bowl, gently toss all ingredients to combine.

17.   **Steakhouse Salad**

Break out this recipe for the hard-core carnivores in your life. It's everything they (and you) love about a steakhouse meal, succulent beef, creamy spinach, and roasted potatoes in salad form. Mushrooms and cherry tomatoes bump up the veg factor, and a light yet full-flavored blue cheese dressing ties it all together.

Active: 25 mins

Total: 25 mins

Yield: Serves 4

Ingredients

10 ounces (4 to 5 small) red potatoes, quartered

2 tablespoons canola oil, divided

1 teaspoon black pepper, divided

1/2 teaspoon kosher salt, divided

1 (8-oz.) beef tenderloin filet

8 ounces cremini mushrooms, quartered

3 garlic cloves, chopped (about 1 1/2 Tbsp.)

1 tablespoon lower-sodium Worcestershire sauce

2 cups cherry tomatoes

1/3 cup low-fat buttermilk

1 tablespoon apple cider vinegar

3 ounces blue cheese, crumbled (about 3/4 cup), divided

8 cups fresh baby spinach (about 6 oz.)

Directions

Preheat oven to 400°F. Toss potatoes with 1 tablespoon of the oil and 1/4 teaspoon each of the pepper and salt on a rimmed baking sheet. Roast potatoes until golden and tender, about 20 minutes, stirring halfway through baking.

Meanwhile, heat remaining 1 tablespoon oil in a heavy skillet over medium-high. Sprinkle beef with 1/4 teaspoon of the pepper and remaining 1/4 teaspoon salt. Sear beef until browned on all sides and a thermometer registers 130°F to 135°F (for medium-rare), about 3 minutes per side, or to desired degree of doneness. Transfer beef to a plate; let rest 5 minutes before slicing.

Return skillet to medium-high. Add mushrooms and garlic, and cook, stirring often, until browned, 2 to 3 minutes. Stir in 2 tablespoons water and Worcestershire, and cook 1 minute. Remove mushroom mixture. Add tomatoes to skillet; cook, stirring occasionally, until blistered, about 4 minutes. Remove from heat.

Stir together buttermilk, vinegar, 1/2 cup of the blue cheese, and remaining 1/2 teaspoon pepper in a large bowl.
Toss spinach in butter milk mixture.

Serve spinach topped with potatoes, beef, mushroom mixture, and tomatoes; sprinkle with remaining 1/4 cup blue cheese.

18.   **Salmon Noodle Bowl**

Omega-3s in salmon and other fatty fish help build more muscle, and more muscle means more calories burned.

Prep: 8 mins

Cook: 20 mins

Total: 28 mins

Yield: Makes 2 servings (serving size: 2 1/4 cups)

Ingredients

4 ounces soba buckwheat noodles or whole-wheat spaghetti

5 ounces asparagus, cut in thirds

Cooking spray
1 (6-oz) salmon fillet, skin off, cut into 8 pieces

1 tablespoon toasted sesame oil

Zest and juice of 1-2 limes (3 TBSP juice)

1/4 teaspoon kosher salt

1/4 teaspoon fresh pepper

4 ounces cucumber, skin on, cut into medium pieces

1/2 small avocado, cut into bite-size pieces

Directions

Cook the noodles in boiling water until soft (about 6 minutes for soba, 8 for spaghetti). Transfer with tongs to a strainer. Add asparagus to same boiling water. Cook until al dente (about 2 minutes); rinse under cold water.

Heat a grill pan or skillet over medium-high heat. Coat lightly with cooking spray. Cook the salmon until cooked through, turning pieces (about 2-3 minutes per side). Reserve.

Make the vinaigrette: Whisk together sesame oil, lime zest and juice, and salt and pepper in a small bowl.
Combine the noodles, asparagus, and vinaigrette in a medium serving bowl.

Add the cucumber and avocado; toss to coat. Just before serving, add salmon. Serve warm or at room temperature, or make up to 4 hours ahead and keep refrigerated in an airtight container.

19.   **Cauliflower and Mushroom Tacos**

Serve these as a vegetarian meal, or with meat-based tacos to mix things up.

Active: 25 mins

Total: 25 mins

Yield: Serves 4

Ingredients

1 cup very thinly sliced red onion

1/4 cup red wine vinegar

1 cup dark Mexican beer (such as Negra Modelo)

1 tablespoon honey

2 tablespoons canola oil

12 ounces cauliflower florets (from 1 head)

6 ounces cremini mushrooms, quartered
1 teaspoon kosher salt

1 teaspoon ground cumin

1/2 teaspoon ancho chile powder

1/4 cup chopped fresh cilantro

8 (6-in.) corn tortillas, warmed

Cotija cheese, pico de gallo, and diced avocado, for garnish

Lime wedges, for serving

Directions

Toss together onion and vinegar in a microwavable dish. Microwave on High for 1 minute; set aside.

Bring beer to a boil in a small saucepan over high; cook until reduced to ½ cup, about 5 minutes. Stir in honey.

Heat oil in a large skillet over high. Add cauliflower and mushrooms. Cook, stirring often, until caramelized and softened, 6 to 8 minutes. Add salt, cumin, and chile powder; cook, stirring often, until fragrant, about 1 minute. Add beer mixture and cilantro; cook, stirring occasionally, until vegetables are tender, about 2 minutes.

Divide vegetable mixture among tortillas. Gently stir onion mixture, and drain any liquid. Top tacos with pickled onion, and garnish with Cotija, pico de gallo, and avocado, if desired. Serve with lime wedges.

20.   Black Bean and Chicken Chilaquiles

Total: 45 mins

Yield: 6 servings

Ingredients

Cooking spray

1 cup thinly sliced onion

5 garlic cloves, minced

2 cups shredded cooked chicken breast

1 (15-ounce) can black beans, rinsed and drained

1 cup fat-free, less-sodium chicken broth

1 (7 3/4-ounce) can salsa de chile fresco (such as El Pato)

15 (6-inch) corn tortillas, cut into 1-inch strips

1 cup shredded queso blanco (about 4 ounces)

Directions

Preheat oven to 450°. Heat a large nonstick skillet over medium-high heat. Coat pan with cooking spray. Add
onion; sauté 5 minutes or until lightly browned. Add garlic; sauté 1 minute. Add chicken; cook 30 seconds. Transfer mixture to a medium bowl; stir in beans. Add broth and salsa to pan; bring to a boil. Reduce heat, and simmer 5 minutes, stirring occasionally. Set aside.

Place half of tortilla strips in bottom of an 11 x 7-inch baking dish coated with cooking spray. Layer half of chicken mixture over tortillas; top with remaining tortillas and chicken mixture. Pour broth mixture evenly over chicken mixture. Sprinkle with cheese. Bake at 450° for 10 minutes or until tortillas are lightly browned and cheese is melted.

21.   **Cioppino**

This technique takes the intimidation out of cooking shellfish. As long as you add each type at its indicated time instead of all at once, you'll end up with delicate, perfectly cooked clams, scallops, shrimp, and mussels. And the flavor of this stew is so rich and deep, you'd never guess it all comes together in about half an hour. This technique takes the intimidation out of cooking shellfish. As long as you add each type at its indicated time instead of all at once, you'll end up with delicate, perfectly cooked clams, scallops, shrimp, and mussels. And the flavor of this stew is so rich and deep, you'd never guess it all comes together in about half an hour.

Active: 35 mins

Total: 35 mins

Yield: Serves 4

Ingredients

1 tablespoon extra-virgin olive oil

1 small yellow onion, sliced

1 small fennel bulb, trimmed and sliced

6 garlic cloves, sliced

1 cup dry white wine

1/4 cup seafood stock

1/4 cup chopped fresh basil, plus more for garnish

1/2 teaspoon crushed red pepper

1 (28-oz.) can no-salt-added whole tomatoes, drained

12 littleneck clams, scrubbed (about 6 oz.)

8 sea scallops (about 8 oz.)

1/2 teaspoon kosher salt

1/2 teaspoon black pepper

8 large peeled and deveined raw shrimp (about 8 oz.)

12 mussels, scrubbed and debearded (about 6 oz.)
2 tablespoon fresh lemon juice

Directions

Heat oil in a large Dutch oven over medium-high; swirl to coat. Add onion and fennel; cook, stirring often, 1 minute. Add garlic; reduce heat to medium, cover, and cook, stirring occasionally, until vegetables are tender, about 8 minutes. Stir in wine, stock, basil, red pepper, and tomatoes; increase heat to medium-high, cover, and bring to a boil. Reduce heat to medium-low, and simmer 10 minutes.

Increase heat to medium-high. Add clams to skillet; cover and cook 2 minutes. Sprinkle scallops with salt and pepper. Add scallops; cover and cook 2 minutes. Add shrimp and mussels; cover and cook until clams and mussels open, about 4 minutes. Discard any unopened shells. Gently stir in lemon juice, and, if desired, sprinkle with basil.

22.   **Harissa Shakshuka With Spinach & Chickpeas**

Bring big flavor to the table, and your diabetic-friendly diet, with this Israeli-inspired dish. Cooking the eggs sunny-side up in a rich tomato sauce imbues them with umami, and a light crumble of feta adds a salty pop to every bite.

Active: 30 mins

Total: 30 mins

Yield: Serves 6

Ingredients

1 tablespoon olive oil

1 cup sliced yellow onion

1 cup chopped red bell pepper

1 cup chopped yellow bell pepper

2 cups lower-sodium marinara sauce

2 tablespoons mild or hot harissa

1 tablespoon chopped fresh oregano

1/2 teaspoon kosher salt

1 (15-oz.) can no-salt-added chickpeas, drained and rinsed

1 (6-oz.) pkg. fresh baby spinach (about 9 cups

6 large eggs

2 ounces feta cheese, crumbled (about ½ cup)

2 tablespoons fresh lemon juice (from one lemon)

Fresh flat-leaf parsley, for garnish

Directions

Heat oil in a large skillet over medium-high. Add onion and bell peppers, and cook, stirring often, until softened, 6 to 8 minutes. Stir in marinara, harissa, oregano, salt, chickpeas, and spinach. Cook, stirring occasionally, until spinach wilts, about 3 minutes.

Make 6 shallow wells in mixture; crack 1 egg into each well. Cover, reduce heat to medium-low, and cook until whites are cooked but yolks are still runny, about 5 minutes.

Remove from heat; sprinkle mixture with feta and lemon juice, and garnish with parsley.

23.   **Italian Garbanzo Salad**

This can be served as a first course or antipasti with Italian food, or as a side to grilled chicken. It's even better the next day over salad greens.

Yield: 8 servings (serving size: about 1 cup)

Ingredients

3 cups finely chopped fennel bulb

2 cups chopped tomato

1 3/4 cups finely chopped red onion

1 cup chopped fresh basil

1/3 cup balsamic vinegar

1 tablespoon olive oil

1 teaspoon freshly ground black pepper

1/4 teaspoon salt

4 garlic cloves, minced

2 (15 1/2-ounce) cans chickpeas (garbanzo beans), rinsed and drained

1/2 cup (2 ounces) crumbled feta cheese

Directions

Combine all ingredients except the cheese in a bowl; toss well. Let stand 30 minutes; sprinkle with cheese.

24. Poached Salmon With Yogurt-Tarragon Sauce

You don't have to worry about drying out fish when it's cooking in liquid! This preparation is so delicate and subtle you can taste the aromatics that are in the cooking liquid, but it doesn't take anything away from the flavor of the salmon. Remember that you're poaching, not boiling: The liquid should be below the boiling point or the fish can get rubbery.

Active: 15 mins
Total: 45 mins

Yield: Serves 4

Ingredients

2 lemons, halved, plus 1 Tbsp. fresh lemon juice

1 cup dry white wine

1 tablespoon whole black peppercorns

2 bay leaves

1/4 cup thinly sliced shallot

1 tablespoon plus ¾ tsp. kosher salt

4 (6-oz.) skinless salmon fillets (1 to 1½ in. thick)

3/4 cup plain whole-milk yogurt

2 tablespoon chopped fresh tarragon, plus more for garnish

1/4 teaspoon black pepper

Directions

Squeeze lemon halves into a high-sided sauté pan or Dutch oven, then add squeezed lemon halves to pan. Add 4 cups water, wine, peppercorns, bay leaves, shallots, and 1 tablespoon of the salt. Bring to a boil over medium-high; cover, reduce heat to medium-low, and simmer 10 minutes. (Adjust heat if needed to make sure liquid is barely steaming with a temperature of about 145°F.)

Add salmon to pan, cover, and cook until a thermometer inserted in fish registers 125°F to 130°F, 10 to 12 minutes. Transfer salmon to a large plate lined with paper towels. Remove and discard any whole peppercorns or bay leaves clinging to fish. Sprinkle fish with ½ teaspoon of the salt. (To serve salmon cold, chill in the refrigerator 30 minutes.)

Stir together yogurt, tarragon, lemon juice, pepper, and remaining ¼ teaspoon salt. If desired, sprinkle fillets with chopped tarragon. Serve with sauce.

25. Spinach-Quinoa Breakfast Salad With Berries And Granola

Berries, granola, yogurt and spinach? Trust us. All the makings of your morning parfait create an unexpected dish with pleasing crunch and pretty pops of color.

Active: 10 mins

Total: 10 mins

Yield: Serves 2
Ingredients

2 teaspoon apple cider vinegar

1 teaspoon pure maple syrup

1/4 teaspoon Dijon mustard

1/4 teaspoon kosher salt

1 tablespoon olive oil

1 (7-oz.) container plain Greek yogurt

3 ounces baby spinach (about 3 cups)

2/3 cup cooked quinoa

2/3 cup quartered fresh strawberries (4 oz.)

1/2 cup fresh blueberries

1/2 cup store-bought almond granola

Directions

Whisk together vinegar, maple syrup, mustard, and salt in a small bowl. Slowly drizzle in oil, whisking constantly, until fully emulsified.

Spread yogurt evenly on 2 plates. Toss together spinach, quinoa, strawberries, blueberries, and half of the dressing in a medium bowl. Divide salad between plates, on top of yogurt. Drizzle with remaining dressing, and sprinkle with granola.

26.   **Crisp Chickpea Slaw**

You need only a little dressing for the slaw because the cabbage releases moisture as it sits. You need only a little dressing for the slaw because the cabbage releases moisture as it sits.

Prep: 10 mins

Total: 10 mins

Yield: Makes 2 servings (serving size: 3 1/2 cups)

Ingredients

1/4 cup fat-free plain yogurt

1 tablespoon cider vinegar

1 tablespoon water

1/4 teaspoon kosher salt

Freshly ground black pepper
1 (15-oz) can low-sodium chickpeas, rinsed and drained

2 1/2 cups sliced packed green cabbage

2 stalks celery, thinly sliced

2 carrots, peeled with a vegetable peeler into strips or thinly sliced, or 2 cups shredded carrots

2 tablespoons sesame seeds, toasted

Directions

In a medium bowl, stir together the yogurt, vinegar, water, salt, and pepper to taste. Add the chickpeas, cabbage, celery, and carrots; toss to combine. Sprinkle with sesame seeds.

Transfer slaw to a plastic food-storage bag or 2 portable containers. Refrigerate at least 4 hours before serving; slaw keeps up to 3 days.

27.   **Egg and Rice Salad to Go**

Any hearty brown rice or brown-rice blend works well in this salad. Great use for leftovers: Any hearty brown rice or brown-rice blend works well in this salad.

Prep: 10 mins

Total: 10 mins

Yield: Makes 1 serving (serving size: about 2.5 cups)
Ingredients

1/2 cup cooked brown rice

1 cup cooked green beans, roughly chopped (3 oz)

1 ripe plum, thinly sliced (3 oz)

2 tablespoons (1/2 oz) chopped walnuts

1 hard-cooked egg, sliced

1 teaspoon sesame oil

2 tablespoons fresh lime juice

1/4 teaspoon kosher salt

Freshly ground black pepper, to taste

Directions

Combine rice, beans, plum, walnuts, and egg in a portable container.

Drizzle with sesame oil, lime juice, salt, and pepper; toss gently to combine. Refrigerate up to 2 days.

28.   **Asian Rice Noodle Salad**

Bonus meal: If you have leftover coleslaw mix, sauté it with a little garlic and ginger and add a protein for a faster-than-takeout mu shu.

Active: 15 mins

Total: 20 mins

Yield: 6 as a side dish

Ingredients

1 Asian brown rice (whole-grain) noodles

1/4 cup low-sodium soy sauce

1 tablespoon rice vinegar

2 tablespoons fresh lime juice
2 teaspoons honey

2 teaspoons toasted sesame oil

1 teaspoon minced fresh ginger

1 clove garlic, minced

3/4 cup fresh cilantro leaves, chopped

3/4 cup chopped salted, dry-roasted peanuts or cashews

2 1/2 cups coleslaw mix

Red pepper flakes, optional

Directions

Cook noodles according to package directions. Drain and transfer to a large bowl to cool. Cut noodles up a bit with kitchen shears or a knife to make them easier to toss.

Whisk together soy sauce, vinegar, lime juice, honey, sesame oil, ginger, and garlic in a small bowl.

Add sauce, cilantro, peanuts, and coleslaw mix to bowl with noodles and toss until well combined. Sprinkle with red pepper flakes to taste, if desired. Serve at room temperature or refrigerate for later.

29.   Chard And Mushroom Butternut Noodles

Enjoying more veggies is probably the No. 1 thing you can do to boost your overall health. While these nutritional superstars can help fend off cancer and other chronic diseases, they can also minimize the effects of aging and contribute to shiny hair and glowing skin. See? Veggies are a win-win! They're also irresistibly delicious, especially when served like "pasta" topped with a hazelnut gremolata for depth of flavor and Parmesan cheese for a hit of umami.

Active: 30 mins

Total: 30 mins

Yield: Serves 4

Ingredients

8 cups spiralized butternut squash (1¼ lb.)

3 tablespoons olive oil, divided

2 tablespoons chopped roasted hazelnuts

1 teaspoon lemon zest, plus 2 Tbsp. fresh juice, divided

2 ounces Parmesan cheese, finely shredded (about ¾ cup), divided

2 teaspoons fresh thyme leaves, divided

1 pound sliced fresh cremini mushrooms

8 cups chopped fresh Swiss chard (from 1 [6-oz.] bunch)

1 tablespoon finely chopped garlic

1 tablespoon unsalted butter

3/4 teaspoon kosher salt

Directions

Preheat oven to 400°F. Toss together butternut squash and 1 tablespoon of the oil on a baking sheet; spread in an even layer. Roast until almost tender, about 8 minutes. Set aside.

While squash roasts, stir together hazelnuts, lemon zest, half of the Parmesan, and 1 teaspoon of the thyme in a small bowl; set aside.

Heat remaining 2 tablespoons oil in a large Dutch oven over medium-high. Add mushrooms; cook, undisturbed, until bottoms start to brown, about 5 minutes. Stir, and continue cooking, stirring occasionally, until golden brown and tender, about 8 minutes. Add chard, garlic, and remaining 1 teaspoon thyme; cook, stirring constantly, until chard wilts, about 2 minutes. Add roasted squash; stir to combine. Remove mixture from heat; stir in lemon juice, butter, salt, and remaining cheese until combined. Divide mixture evenly among 4 bowls; sprinkle with hazelnut mixture. Serve immediately.

30.   **Sausage & Kale Strata**

This take on a classic casserole is hearty but won't weigh your guests down. Gruyère, sausage, and kale is a great seasonal combo; swapping in wholegrain bread adds extra nutrition and staying power. Assembling everything the night before gives the bread the chance to soak up the liquid.

Active: 20 mins

Total: 1 hr 30 mins
Yield: Serves 12

Ingredients

1 tablespoons olive oil

1 pound mild or hot Italian turkey sausage, casings removed

1 cup chopped yellow onion

2 (4-oz.) bunches Lacinato kale, stemmed and thinly sliced

2 cups 2% reduced-fat milk

1/2 teaspoon dry mustard

1/2 teaspoon kosher salt

1/4 teaspoon black pepper

8 large eggs

1 (16-oz.) hearty whole-grain bread loaf, cut into 1-in. cubes

Cooking spray

4 ounces Gruyère cheese, shredded (about 1 cup), divided

Directions

Heat oil in a large nonstick skillet over medium-high. Add sausage and onion; cook, stirring often, until sausage is browned and onion is tender, 6 to 8 minutes. Stir in kale, and cook until wilted, about 1 minute. Remove from heat, and let cool 5 minutes.

Whisk together milk, mustard, salt, pepper, and eggs in a large bowl.

Combine bread cubes and sausage mixture in a 9x13-inch baking dish coated with cooking spray. Pour milk mixture evenly over bread mixture, pressing gently to submerge bread in liquid. Sprinkle evenly with cheese; cover with lightly greased (with cooking spray) aluminum foil, and chill at least 8 hours or up to overnight.

Remove dish from refrigerator; let stand 30 minutes. Preheat oven to 350°F. Bake in preheated oven, covered, for 30 minutes. Uncover and bake until lightly browned and set, about 15 minutes. Let stand 10 minutes before serving.

Prep this the day before and sleep in a little the next morning!

Conclusion

To conclude, Optavia diet program is result oriented and well-balanced weight loss program, and has gained so much of popularity in the industry over the past 45 years. It is very effective and you will start seeing the results in the first week itself. The diet program has assisted millions of individuals in losing and controlling their weight. The portion controlled meals are convenient to consume, and you can get over the burden of grocery shopping and food preparation. You can reheat the food just before consuming that is all, you do not have to do anything else. Stop thinking. Start taking action and lose weight.

Meal replacements are at the center of this low-calorie diet. This may appeal to some since it largely eliminates the need for most planning, shopping, and food prep. However, individuals who prefer freshly prepared food and variety in their diet are not likely to find the program sustainable or realistic.

The Optavia Diet does address more health concerns, lifestyle conditions, and age groups than most other commercial diet programs, but special populations, particularly those with diabetes, should always consult a physician before making changes to diet.

Detox Revolution 2021

Table of Contents

Introduction

Thank you for downloading my book. Because you downloaded it you are clearly looking for more information on detox cleanses and how they work, how they can help you to drop weight, smooth out those wrinkles and help you feel much more refreshed and healthy. But why do we need to detox? Doesn't the human body already do it for us naturally?

Well, yes it does to a certain degree but it can only be effective if your body isn't overloaded with toxins and pollutants and that's where the trouble lies these days. While technology and science have brought no end of improvements to our lives, they have also filled the air we breathe with pollutants and so many of us are finding that we are taking in more toxins than our bodies can possibly remove.

Toxins come from everywhere – in the air we breathe, the water we drink and the ground we walk on. They come from the many synthetic materials that we use or wear on a daily basis and they come from the food we eat. You could argue that you eat a healthy diet but you would be shocked to know just how many toxins are laced through the meat you eat, the seafood, even the vegetables. And, for those who eat a "junk" diet, well, your bodies really are overloaded.

Would it really surprise you to know that your food is laced with chemicals, pesticides, metals? Processed food is especially bad for this but it's also in the water you drink as well. There are more chronic illnesses in evidence now than there ever has been and because of the sheer number of different toxins passing into the body every day, it's become impossible for us to remove them naturally.

With this book, my aim is to show you why you need to detox and how to do it safely. I will tell you what builds up in the body, where it comes from and how to remove it with some very simple steps, steps that anyone can take. I will tell you what foods you should eat and what you shouldn't and I will also give you a couple of recipes to take away with you and try. So, without any further waiting, let's dive in and see what's what.

Chapter 1:

What is Detoxification?

Detox is short for detoxification and it is a natural process whereby the body removes toxins from our blood and our organs. Toxins are, to put it simply, poisons. Anything that can cause harm to the body tissues is a toxin, including waste products that come from cell activity – waste products like ammonia, homocysteine, and lactic acid. Add to that the man-made toxins we are exposed to on a daily basis and it's easy to see how our bodies can become overloaded.

In order to eliminate toxins from the body, the intestines, liver, kidneys, skin, blood, lungs, and our lymphatic systems all work together to turn harmful toxins into harmless compounds that can be eliminated out of the body, through sweat, urine and bowel elimination.

Because of the sheer number of toxins we are exposed to our bodies are struggling to remove them efficiently. If the body cannot use what we ingest nutritionally or eliminate it naturally, it will remain in our blood and lymphatic systems, eventually moving into body tissues, and staying put.

Detoxification is the process of cleansing the body of these toxins and giving your system a boost it so desperately needs.

What is a Toxin?

Toxins are any compounds that affect cell function or cell structure in an adverse manner and includes:

- Heavy Metals – Mercury, lead, aluminum – accumulate in the kidneys, brain and immune system

- Liver Toxicants – Alcohol, drugs, pesticides, toxic chemicals, food additives – constant exposure can cause severe liver damage

- Microbial Toxins – Toxins absorbed by yeast and bacteria that lives in the intestines – can cause serious disruptions to normal bodily functions

- Products of the Breakdown of Protein Metabolism – ammonia and urea – can overload the kidneys, especially if you eat too much protein

Every day we are exposed to herbicides, pesticides, food additives, solvents and so many other toxins and, most of the time, we don't even realize it. It's not like you know you are breathing in or ingesting these toxins because you can see or taste them – if you did, you wouldn't do it.

Asthma, chronic fatigue, lupus, fibromyalgia, migraines, and multiple sclerosis can all be attribute to constant exposure to these toxins. Studies have shown that people who suffer from any of these have experienced a reversal of their symptoms after they have been through a total cleansing detoxification process.

A full detox process will improve your health in so many ways by:

- Removing heavy metals – including mercury and lead

- Detoxifying – the liver, kidneys, blood and other body organs

- Recharging your immune system – through introducing powerful antioxidants into your body

- Replenishing friendly bacteria – especially the most important ones in the intestines

10 Signs That Your Liver Needs a Detox

You already know by now that your liver is one of the most powerful organs in your body and, next to the heart is one of the hardest working. Your liver has two jobs – detoxifying your body and working as a digestive organ. In today's modern world, most of us have a liver that is over-worked and cannot cope. Unfortunately, most of us don't listen to the signs so the following 10 signs should help you to realize that your liver is crying out to you for relief:

- Bloating around the abdomen
- Pain around the liver area
- Too much belly or abdominal fat
- You struggle to digest fatty foods
- You have had your gallbladder out
- You suffer with acid reflux or heartburn
- You have liver spots on your skin
- You sweat excessively and overheat quickly
- You have acne, rosacea or dry blotchy and itchy skin
- You put on weight unexpectedly and can't lose it even on a

calorie controlled diet There are a number of other signs that will give it away as well, including:

- High blood pressure
- Fatigue
- High triglycerides and cholesterol
- Depression
- Mood swings
- Sleep apnea
- Snoring

- Yellow fatty lumps around the eyes

These are all signs that your liver is struggling and that you need to detox, change your diet and shake up your lifestyle in order for your liver to heal. What these signs are telling you is that your liver is blocked up with unhealthy fat, if it's extreme, it's called fatty liver disease. The cells in your liver that are used as filters become swollen up with fat and cannot filter the rubbish out. Remember that the blood is filtered through the liver, cleaned out and sent back to the heart. If you don't clean your liver out, you are sending toxic blood back up to your heart that can cause damage to the cardiovascular system, the immune system and it can cause rapid aging.

How Does Fatty Liver Happen?

There are two ways – the first is through alcohol and the second is through diet. People who don't drink can get NAFD – Non Alcoholic Fatty Liver Disease and this is generally attributed to following a diet that is high in carbohydrates and processed or sugary foods.

What Else?

As we already talked about earlier, there are such high levels of toxins all around these days that we can't escape them. They are on our food in the form of pesticides, in our water, in food preservatives, electromagnetic radiation and heavy metals. They come into our blood through the food, the air, even through home cleaning and personal care products. They move in to the bowel, the kidneys, the liver, fat tissue and the lymphatic system and they build up, stopping our bodies from taking in the nutrients, proteins, carbohydrates and using them effectively. It even reduces that amount of oxygen in your blood and puts you into a state of low energy, susceptible to disease.

Because the liver is working so hard to try to filter these toxins out, it can't do all its others jobs, resulting in a weight gain and a struggle to lose it again.

REMEMBER

Your skin is the single biggest organ in your body and what goes on it goes through it. The simple rule of thumb is this – if you wouldn't eat it, don't put it on your skin. Even those products that are labeled as organic might have used toxins in the preserving process so try to go for those with essential preservatives.

If you can make your own skin products using coconut oil, organic shea butter, olive oil, jojoba oil and essential oils.

Be aware that lots of things we take for granted these days emit electromagnetic fields, such as cordless phones, mobile phones, Wi-Fi, airplanes and x-rays. When you are sleeping, keep all electronic things at least 8 feet away from you, if not in another room.

The next thing you must do is look at your diet and eliminate the foods that are harming your liver. Get rid of processed foods, those that are high in sugars and simple carbohydrates. Eat more raw food, such as vegetables and fruits and, if you do cook, don't overcook foods. Get rid of your microwave, as this does nothing but destroy anything good that was in the food.

Make the switch to high quality oils, such as olive or coconut and eliminate the lower quality oils.

Don't eat animal products that are not grass-fed or free range.

If you have at least three of the symptoms listed above, cut alcohol out of your diet altogether.

Add supportive foods to your diet – lots of brightly colored fruits and vegetables and dark leafy greens. At least 30- 40% of your diet should be raw vegetables and fruits. These are useful because they have living enzymes in them, as well as vitamin C, phyto-nutrients and natural antibiotics. If you don't like eating them raw, juice them or add them to a smoothie.

You should also try to eat foods that are naturally fermented, such as sauerkraut, apple cider vinegar, cultured vegetables and yogurt. The other important nutrients that your body needs are:

- **Vitamin K** – from dark leafy vegetables

- **Arginine** – legumes, oats, carob, walnuts, seeds and wheat germ. These help the liver to detoxify ammonia

- **Antioxidants** – raw carrot, beetroot, celery, apple, pear, dandelion juices and green drinks that are made contain spirulina and chlorella. Also found in fresh kiwi and citrus fruits

- **Selenium** – Brazil nuts, brown rice, kelp, seafood, molasses, garlic, whole grains, onion, wheat germ

- **Methionine** – Legumes, fish, eggs, onion, garlic, seeds, meat

- **Essential fatty acids** – cod liver oil seafood, fish oil. Seafood can be frozen, fresh or canned and includes salmon, sardines, mackerel, trout, tuna, blue mussels, mullet, herring, calamari and blue eye cod. Avocado, raw nuts, seeds, whole grains, legumes, green vegetables, such as spinach, kale, beet greens. Eggplant, cold pressed seed and vegetable oils, fresh ground seeds, evening primrose oil, starflower oil and blackcurrant seed oil. EFAs are needed to keep the cells in the body healthy and you need to consume them in plentiful amounts to keep your liver functioning properly. This is why low fat diets are generally not good for weight control, health and liver function.

- **Natural sulfur** – eggs, onions, garlic, leeks, shallots, broccoli, cabbage, cauliflower, Brussels sprouts

Finally, in order to help your liver get back to tip top condition you should use supportive nutrients and herbs. The B complex vitamins are important for liver function, as are natural beta-carotenes, and vitamins C and E. Globe artichokes; milk thistle, dandelion and turmeric are also good for helping the liver.

What is a Detox Cleanse?

Most of us assume that detox is primarily a treatment for dependence on drugs or alcohol. However, a detox cleanse is also used as a method of losing weight, clearing the skin and generally improving health. A detox cleanse is a short-term way of rebooting your life, of removing all those chemicals and toxins from your body and giving you a clean slate to start over with.

Detox diets are not long-term solutions. If you were to follow a detox diet for any longer than a few days your body would be deprived of essential nutrients and you would not be getting balance of the food groups that you need for optimum health.

You can follow a detox diet for up to one week but you must then move on to a healthy diet. There is no harm in repeating the detox on a regular basis – some people kick start their bodies with a one week cleanse and then do a three day cleanse once a month afterwards – this will not harm you provided you are eating a sensible diet in between times.

A detox cleanse will:

- Drastically reduce the amount of chemicals that you ingest

- Place more importance on the foods that contain the nutrients, vitamins and essential antioxidants that your body needs to detoxify itself naturally

- Contain food groups that are high in water content and fiber, both of which help to draw out and eliminate the toxins – this works because by eating more fiber and drinking more water, the frequency of urination and bowel movements you experience will increase.

- Help to prevent chronic diseases. Toxins that we encounter in the environment are responsible for so many neurological diseases, cancers, strokes, heart disease, and so many more. While our bodies do naturally detox, they can't cope when they are overloaded so a detox gives us a boost and helping hand.

• Enhances your immune system function. If your immune system has been compromised, you are significantly more likely to catch flu, colds and other viruses, which affect your productivity and your quality of life. Detoxing on a regular basis helps build up strength in the immune system and helps to fight off infection.

• Drop those pounds. A healthy body has a natural ability to burn off excess fat but an overload of toxins stops that from working. As we all know, a number of chronic diseases are linked with weight gain, including heart disease, diabetes and high blood pressure. Detoxing removes the toxins in the fat cells and increases your metabolism rate.

• Slows down premature aging. Heavy metals and free radicals are partly responsible for rapid aging and detox will eliminate those from the body. This means your body will increase more nutrients, including vitamins and antioxidants that help to fight off oxidative stress.

• Improve your quality of life. Put simply, if our bodies are overloaded with toxins, they will not function as they should. You may experience pain in your joints, a lack of energy, trouble sleeping, headaches and problems digesting your food. Detoxing can improve your memory function and ease depression as well.

• Increase your energy. A detox will give you more physical, mental and emotional energy and you will sleep much better.

• Improve your skin quality. Toxins cause acne, weak hair and weak nails as well as making us look pale and ill. Regular detox cleansing will improve all of that and give you back a healthy glow.

• Improve your emotional and mental clarity. This will allow you to deal with more, make better decisions and think much clearer. You will also see things differently and won't be prone to seeing a small problem as something that is insurmountable.

• Restore the balance to your body. Overloads of toxins and bad foods stop your hormonal, digestive and nervous systems from working together in harmony and make you ill. Detoxing restores the balance.

Chapter 2:

Who Shouldn't Try a Detox Cleanse?

While detox cleanses are generally safe, you should consult your doctor first. People who definitely should not undertake a detox cleanse are pregnant or nursing women, young children, or anyone who has a disease of the kidneys or liver. This is also not intended to be used as a way of treating alcohol or drug related dependencies – these must be treated in the correct manner.

If you suffer with a persistent cough, pain in the muscles, indigestion, or insomnia, do not assume that it's because your body is overloaded with toxins. It may well be but you do need to see a doctor first to ensure that there is nothing more serious going on.

Side Effects of a Detox Cleanse

The single most common side effect of a detox cleanse is a headache and this can last for a couple of days. This is mainly down to a withdrawal from caffeine. To avoid this, before you start a detox cleanse, gradually decrease how much caffeine you drink so it isn't such a shock to the system.

Other side effects can cause bad diarrhea, which will lead to a loss of electrolytes and dehydration. If you eat too much fiber, the opposite can occur – chronic constipation. To avoid this you must drink plenty of fluids. You may experience tiredness, hunger, irritability and an outbreak of acne but these are extreme cases.

For these reasons, you should try to start your detox cleanse on a weekend or take some time off work. It's only for a few days and you will feel so much better afterwards as your body clears the rubbish out and makes way for good health.

How to Deal With the Symptoms of a Detox

Not everyone will feel great to start with on a detox and, if you find that you need a bit of a push to get past a sticking point, these tips will help you:

- **Drink**. I already said above to make sure you are drinking enough water to maintain your hydration levels. This also helps to stop you becoming constipated. A detox can involve a high level of fiber, which can stop you from going so get drinking!

- **Sweat** – Toxins in our bodies are removed in three ways – through the digestive tract, through the lungs and through the skin. Work up a sweat through doing some light exercise and the toxins will exit your body through your pores. As well as that, your lymph fluid will get moving again. You could also use a wet or dry sauna or a steam room to produce the same results.

- **Have a Massage** – massages are good for sore muscles but they also stimulate the lymph fluid and get it flowing again. Your lymphatic system is vital to get rid of waste that the body doesn't need. Blood and lymph fluid circulation can help you to recover from the symptoms of detox a lot quicker. You can also add Epsom salts to your bath and soak in it for half an hour after dry brushing dead skin cells off.

- **Find a Substitute** - cravings are tough to deal with but instead of heading for the chocolate, pick a piece of fruit or a handful of nuts, something from the list of foods that you are allowed to eat. If you really do crave chocolate, add some raw cacao to a smoothie. If you crave salt, add kelp seasoning to food.

If you are missing fat, eat an avocado or add it to your smoothie, with a spot of coconut oil. In time, you can train your brain to look for healthy alternatives to processed foods.

- **Rest** – A couple of days in to your detox cleanse, you may start feeling a little fatigued. Don't try to fight it, you will only feel worse. Respect your limits and listen to your body. If you are tires, rest, sneak a ten-minute power nap on your lunch break if you can. Give it a couple of days and you will have so much energy you won't know what to do with it.

- **Breathe** – You can help to release toxins by learning deep breathing and yoga exercises. Also, deep belly breathing will help to stimulate your lymph flow as well as calming your body and your mind

5 Reasons You Need a Detox Cleanse

When we talk about detox, many of us automatically envisage hunger, deprivation, weird and wonderful juices and drinks. We may wonder if it is worth all the effort and the suffering. You don't need to suffer with a detox cleanse – yes, you may get a headache and you may get a touch of diarrhea but only if you don't do it right, if you jump straight into it without preparing yourself first.

You might also be asking yourself if you really need a detox cleanse so, if you are one of those take a look at these 5 reasons why you do need one – I bet you can identify with at least one of them:

1. You have FLC Syndrome

FLC stands for, to put it bluntly, Feel Like Crap. When you wake up you don't feel awake. You have no energy; you drag yourself out of the bed and through your morning routine without any sense of joy or vitality. Think about this– do you suffer with fatigue, allergies, digestive problems, brain fog, headaches? If you do then barring any other medical issues, a detox can help you to get rid of that FLC syndrome.

2. You struggle to lose weight and/or keep it off

Yes, I know, everyone will tell you that losing weight and keeping it off is nothing more than decreasing your calories and increasing your exercise. OK, so that can help but it isn't the whole story. For instance, did you know that not all calories are equal? That the calories in flour and sugar are totally different to other calories? These calories trigger overeating and a type of addiction. They raise your insulin levels and increase inflammation in the body, that's why you store fat in your belly, and you never feel full up. A detox removes those calories from the equation and teaches you a completely new way of eating that helps you drop the pounds and keep them off while feeling full and eating less.

3. You get really bad cravings for sugar and carbs

Flour and sugar are addictive; there is no two ways about it. It's been proven time and time again. Yet, are we not quick to accuse an overweight person of being lazy? Add to this that most of the foods you eat containing sugar and flour are processed and you get an additional overload of chemicals and toxins that you really don't need. But it is these toxins that cause the cravings and a detox cleanse removes that instantly.

Just as an aside, it may interest you to know that sugar is more than 8 times more addictive than a drug like cocaine and using sheer willpower to lose weight simply will not work. You need to detox your body and train yourself to understand that you do not need sugar or any processed floury sugary foods whatsoever.

4. You have never done a detox in your entire life

Most of us haven't but we should. It's only a few days here and there, nothing in the grand scheme of things. Just a few days to fill your body with clean food and get rid of the buildup of toxins. If you think you feel healthy now, wait until you have been through a detox cleanse and then tell me what healthy feels like!

5. Your body needs a break

And so do you. The way we live our lives these days is not conducive to good health – we sleep too little, we eat too much junk, we don't exercise enough and we get stressed out. And we don't take enough time out for us. One of the best ways to reset your life is a detox cleanse. You are only a few days away from feeling the best you have ever felt, a few days away from being happy and healthy again.

Five Ways to Detox

If you want to lose weight, lose the wrinkles, and feel great again, you need to undergo a detox. Choose from these five ways to kick start your life again:

1. Go cold turkey

This is the only way to handle a true physiological addiction. If you are addicted to junk foods, the only way to get them out of your system completely is to stop it. Go on a 3, 5 or 7-day detox and reset the hormones and neurotransmitters in your body, Get rid of the toxins, eliminate cravings and increase your metabolism. I'm not just talking about food that you eat either. Think about what you drink. Did you know that the latte you grab on the way into work has more sugar in it than a can of soda? All that does is makes you want to eat.

Check your labels – cut out anything that has Trans fats, hydrogenated fats, and monosodium glutamate (MSG). In fact, don't eat anything that comes in a box, a packet, even a can and stick to eating whole fresh foods. The best way to detox quickly is to eliminate grains from your diet for a week and cut out sugar and alcohol.

2. Power up with protein

Protein is the best thing you can eat, at every single meal, most importantly at breakfast. Protein helps to balance out the cravings for sugar so start the day with eggs or a good protein smoothie. Eat seeds, nuts, fish, chicken or eggs at every meal. Make sure you use organic grass fed meats and butters.

3. Don't limit the good carbs

Vegetables contain carbs Fruit contains carbs although a lot of fruits are high in sugars as well. Avoid starchy carbs and fill up of greens – kale, spinach, beet greens, broccoli, cauliflower, and collards. Eat asparagus, mushrooms, zucchini, onions, green beans, tomatoes and fennel. Cut out potatoes, squash, beets – just for 1 week and see how it makes you feel. I guarantee you will lose weight, you will look younger and you will feel great and you will never want to go back to the way you used to eat.

4. Eat fat not sugar

For so many years we have been told that fat is bad for us but now, at long last, nutritionists and doctors have finally understood the difference between good fat and bad fat and just how important the first one is in our diets. Good fat fills you up and evens out the glucose in your blood. You don't get the insulin spikes or the sugar highs and lows. Eat oily fish, butter, nuts, seeds, olive oil, avocadoes, all excellent sources of omega 3 and 6 fats. And they are not called essential for nothing!

5. Forget willpower, use friend power instead

If you are looking to lose weight and feel great then forget willpower. It will not work. What will work is doing a detox cleanse with a friend. You have the right kind of support and the push you need to keep going and you can compare results!

Detox for Fast Weight Loss

Let's answer one of the most common questions asked – do detox diets really work? Do they live up to all that hype? The answer is yes, they do work, but only if you follow them correctly. Most detox diets are short – between 3 and 21 days and they are highly calorie restricted. They cut out the fast food, the processed food, the alcohol, sugar, caffeine and some of them will even eliminate wheat, dairy and meat. Most of them are heavily focused on vegetables and fruit, sometimes in their raw form and sometimes in a juice or a smoothie.

You can lose a significant amount of weight doing a detox but you must keep one thing in mind. Most of the initial weight loss will be water and if you go straight back to your old eating habits afterwards, the weight will pile back on. You should use a detox cleansing diet as the starting point of a new way of life, a new way of eating, although you can use one just to drop a dress size beer a big event if you want.

One thing that all detox diets contain is cleansing elements. They contain fluid and fiber, both of which help eliminate metabolic waste out of the body. Certain herbs and nutritional supplements may be included to help stimulate the enzymes in the liver that break the toxins down. When it comes down to the wire, we all know, deep down, that a whole food diet is better than a juice fast but you can start your regime with a juice diet and ease yourself in to a whole food diet. Whole foods help to improve your metabolism, support your liver and your colon and you can lose weight easily without having to starve yourself for days.

Detox diets are also very good for helping to identify the foods that are taking their energy, food allergies and to help cut the cravings for bad foods. The real benefit to any diet comes a couple of weeks after starting, which is when the fat loss really begins to start happening. A detox diet, followed by a whole food diet is going to have more effect than a 3-day detox followed by you going back to your normal eating habits.

What I am going to give you now is a way to drop a quick 5 lbs. to lighten the load a bit – without starving yourself! The following meal plan will fill you up with metabolism boosting carbs, helping you to burn off fat while you stay fuller for longer. Follow the plan for 5 days and drop 5 lbs. You can extend it to 7 days but no more.

Either eat these meals every day for 5 days or make up your own meal plan using similar ingredients; this is just to start you off.

Breakfast Banana Shake Ingredients:

- 1 large banana
- 12 oz. 1% milk – low fat
- 2 tsp honey
- ½ cup ice

Preparation

- Chop the banana
- Put the ice in the blender, followed by all other ingredients
- Blend until smooth

Lunch

Pecan Crusted Goats Cheese Salad, Pomegranate Vinaigrette Ingredients:

- 4 oz. polenta, cut into slices about ½ inch thick
- 1 oz. goats cheese
- 1 tbsp. pecans, chopped
- 2 tbsp. pomegranate juice
- 1 tsp olive oil
- 1 tsp Dijon mustard
- 3 cups fresh spinach
- ½ cup carrot, shredded

Preparation

- Heat up a nonstick pan over a medium heat. Spray cooking oil over the polenta and put them in the pan, cook for 5 minutes. Turn the slices and cook for a further 5 minutes

- Make a patty out of the goats cheese and coat it with the chopped pecans

- Mix the pomegranate juice, mustard and oil together in a small bowl; which to combine thoroughly

- Put the spinach and carrot onto a serving plate, top with the polenta and the cheese

- Sprinkle vinaigrette over and enjoy!

Dinner

Black Bean, Brown Rice, Avocado and Chicken Wrap
Ingredients

- ½ tsp salt

- ¼ tsp black pepper

- 1 1/3 cups black beans, low sodium, drained and properly rinsed

- 1 tsp chili powder

- ½ tsp cumin

- ¼ tsp chili flakes

- 8 oz. chicken breast, grilled and sliced

- 4 whole wheat wraps

- 1 1/3 cup brown rice, cooked

- 1 small shredded carrot

- ½ avocado, stone removed and diced

- 1 Roma tomato, seeds removed and chopped

- Hot sauce – optional

Preparation

- Mix the first 6 ingredients together and toss
- Put a wrap flat on a clean surface
- Spoon 1/3 cup of rice on the bottom of it and add 1/3 cup bean mix, 2 oz. chicken and ¼ cup carrot
- Add 1 tbsp. of avocado and 2 tbsp. tomato
- Seal the wrap up, cut in half and serve straight away; season with hot sauce if desired

Snack

Greek Yoghurt Parfait Ingredients

- 3 cups of fat free plain Greek yogurt
- 1 tsp vanilla extract
- 4 tsp honey
- 28 segments of clementine
- ¼ cup unsalted dry roasted shelled and chopped pistachios

Preparation

- Mix the yogurt and the honey together
- Spoon 1/3 cup of the mix into each of 4 parfait glasses
- Add ½ tsp honey to the top, with 5 sections of clementine and ½ tbsp. nuts
- Add another 1/3 cup of the honey and yogurt mixture on to the top of each
- Add a further ½ tsp of honey, 2 more segments of clementine and ½ tbsp. nuts
- Serve straight away

All-Day Drink

Fat Flushing Cooler Ingredients

- 8 cups of brewed green tea

- As many slices of lime, orange and lemon as you want

Preparation

- Pour the green tea into a pitcher

- Add the fruit slices

- Drink it warm or refrigerate and serve over ice

- You can drink a pitcher of this every day

Detox for Anti-Aging

To detox your skin to prevent rapid aging, you do not have to spend a small fortune on creams or plastic surgery. The best way to detox your skin and give you back that youthful complexion and glow is to eat the right foods. You need foods that are full of antioxidant nutrients and vitamins to give your cells a helping hand in absorbing the nutrients. This, in turn, eliminated the toxins that are aging and drying your skin. The following is a list of the best foods for your skin and should be on your shopping list:

Red Peppers

Red peppers contain more than 9 times as much carotene and two times as much vitamin C than green peppers do, evidenced by their rich bright color. They also taste nicer! Red peppers contain folate, one of the best antioxidants for antiaging, along with vitamin A, which helps to stop the harmful UV rays from causing damage to your skin. They are also full of other antioxidants, which help to keep you healthy

Brown Rice

Brown rice is not only tastier and more textured than white rice, it also has more vitamin B1, which helps to regulate circulation, keeping it healthy. Good blood circulation helps to stop the loss of skin elasticity and also stops the skin from wrinkling. It has more fiber than any other type of rice because it has not been removed from its husk, making it one of the best foods for detoxing.

Berries

Berries may be small but they are capable of magic. One of the things they can do is prevent cellulite form forming by boosting your circulation and the flow of blood and lymph fluids. All of that stops your skin from dimpling in certain areas of the body and the antioxidants in the berries plump the cells out. This also stops your skin from looking worn out and tired.

Leafy Greens

Especially the darker ones. Leafy green vegetables are packed full of anti-oxidants, especially a coenzyme called Q10. No doubt you have heard of this, as it is an ingredient in many skin creams. However, you don't need to go to that expense when you can get the same coenzyme in its natural form by eating broccoli, kale and spinach, all of which are a lot cheaper than the latest anti-aging cream. Q10 helps cell to grow and, as we age, our bodies stop producing so much, thus needing a bit of a helping hand.

Quinoa

This is a pseudo-cereal that tastes similar to couscous or rice. It is one of the more expensive grains but is one of life's super foods, full of protein and great for anti-aging detoxification.

Lean Protein

If you tend to buy fatty cuts of meat, swap them out for lean cuts. Lean meat contains a lower level of saturated fat than regular cuts and this saves your body all the extra work of digesting and processing the excess. Lean proteins include chicken, oily fish and turkey, which all help to repair cells. Oily fish is good for boosting your collagen levels and is packed full of omega-3 essential fatty acids.

Cinnamon

Strangely, cinnamon stops the growth of bacteria and boosts brain function, as well helping to lower cholesterol, triglyceride and glucose levels. A good all-rounder, cinnamon cuts down damage to the cells, which helps your skin to stay looking younger.

Mediterranean Herbs

Herbs like oregano, parsley, rosemary and basil are all excellent ingredients for an anti-aging detox diet. Oregano is especially good as it has more than 20 times the potency of antioxidants than most other herbs.

Eggs

Eggs are a complete protein, which makes then an excellent choice for helping with the effects of aging. They contain vitamins A, B12, D and K as well as lutein, which also help to maintain the health of your eyes.

Walnuts and Cashews

Both of these contain copper, which, in low levels, can actually stop your hair from going grey prematurely. Copper helps the body to produce melanin, which is what gives your hair its color.

Fresh Fish

Fish is well known for its health benefits and you will always find them on any anti-aging detox diet. Fish like tilapia, salmon, sardines and trout contain very high levels of omega-3 and vitamins that help to keep you looking younger. Fish are also good for helping the cardiovascular system and promoting healthy eyes.

Herbal Teas

Herbal tea has long been known for helping to detox and improve skin health. Green tea in particular is one of the best but all herbal teas help to clean out your system, and push antioxidants through which help to fight off the damage done by free radicals. Tea is easily accepted by the body because it can extract the nutrients that help fight bacteria, heal up wounds, skin breaks, and cleanse those toxins right out.

Citrus Fruits

Citrus fruits such as lemons, limes, oranges and grapefruit can make you look younger because they are loaded with antioxidants. They help to flush the organs out, like your intestines, and will break down and remove bacteria and toxins. They also have high water content and, as you know by now, a detox is a waste of time if you don't keep your body hydrated. Citrus also has fat burning properties, thus making you look younger and helping you to burn off the unwanted pounds.

Pineapples

Pineapples are excellent parts of an anti-aging detox diet because they contain bromelain. This is a collection of enzymes that help to improve the health of your digestive system. The cleaner you colon is, the healthier you will feel and the younger you will look.

All of these foods will help to boost your immune system and keep it healthy, keeping you regular and reducing the chance of an infection. Tired and old looking skin happens because your skin is desperately trying to detox your body and this causes the spots, wrinkles and bags under the eyelids. Change your diet, change your life, it's a simple as that.

The next chapter is going to look at two different methods of detox – short and long-term, along with a few tips on how to detox safely.

How to Detox

Short-term

There are three main ways that you can do a short-term detox but, for all three methods, the real emphasis here is on short!

Fruit Detox

The fruit detox is a good way to detox without going hungry. Amongst the obvious health benefits of eating fruit, this also helps to increase your energy levels, lose weight, and could cut down on your chances of a stroke. You can do this eating just one type of fruit (make it your favorite one) or by eating a variety of different fruits. You must not go more than 7 days on a fruit detox diet!

For best results:

Choose citrus fruits such as oranges, grapefruits, lemons, tangerines, mandarins and limes. These contain excellent detoxifying properties and go well either on their own or combined with other fruits.

Try a grape detox. Grapes contain something called reservatrol (particularly red or black grapes) that can help to prevent blood clots and fight cancer and diabetes. They also contain high levels of vitamin C and potassium. For a maximum of 3-5 days, eat ONLY grapes and nothing else.

Liquid Detox

For 2-3 days eat nothing, just drink water, fruit juice, tea (green or black tea is best), vegetable juices and/or protein smoothies. These work by cutting down the amount of calories you are taking in and can help to flush out toxins from your body.

For best results:

Drink fruit and vegetable juices so that your body is receiving adequate nourishment, vitamins, and minerals. Make your own from fresh fruits and vegetables rather than drinking shop bought ones as these contain sugars and other ingredients you don't want.

If you choose a liquid detox, you will have to seriously rethink your diet if your goal is weight loss. Otherwise, as soon as you go back to a normal diet all the weight will go back on.

Fruit and Vegetable Detox

Instead of just fruits, eat a variety of vegetables as well for 7 days. Both contain minerals, vitamins and other vital nutrients that your body requires for optimum health. Eat a wide range to make sure you get all you need.

For best results:

- Eat beans, such as kidney and black beans, apples, blueberries, artichokes and soybeans for fiber
- Eat carrots, lima beans, cooked greens, sweet potatoes, ordinary potatoes, and bananas for potassium
- Eat strawberries, kiwi, cauliflower, tomato, kale, Brussels Sprouts, bell peppers, mango, and oranges for vitamin C
- Eat melons, cooked spinach, oranges, asparagus and black-eyed peas for folate
- Eat coconut, olives and avocadoes for good fats

Long-term

Change Your Diet

Swap processed foods for organic meat and organic produce. The fruit and vegetables you buy in a supermarket are grown using chemicals, herbicides, and pesticides while organic produce contains only natural fertilizers and pesticides. Organic meats are raised on natural grass and contain none of the chemicals, antibiotics, and growth hormones that are normally fed to animals.

For best results:

- Make sure everything you eat is organic – look for a green USDA Certified Organic Seal on packaging

- Only eat grass-fed animal products, such as meat, butter, milk, eggs, cheese, etc.

- Drink plenty of water, at least 2-4 liters every day. As well as keeping you hydrated, it flushes out the toxins from your kidneys. You don't have to drink plain water if you really can't face it, add fruit and vegetables to it – particularly citrus fruit as this helps to boost your fat-burning properties. Later, I will give you some recipes for flavored waters that will help you get through your day much easier

- Cut the alcohol. It has now been shown that alcohol is linked to cancer, so cut down to one glass a night, no more. Don't be tempted to cut it out all week and then binge on a Friday or Saturday night – that is far worse than drinking all week.

- Cut out sugar, which you will do if you remove processed foods from your diet anyway.

Detox Tips

- Try and detox with a friend for support

- Eat slowly. Chewing your food thoroughly helps with digestion and gives your body a chance to process all that it is receiving

- Don't forget the exercise. Stick to light exercise during a detox, such as Pilates or yoga.

- Rest up properly. Make sure you get sufficient sleep every night and add in afternoon naps if necessary.

- Go for a massage, it will help the toxins to come out of your body much quicker

Warnings

Do not continue past the 7-10 days mark on a fasting detox. Long term fasting can do irreparable damage Research your detox diet thoroughly before undertaking it; speak to your doctor if necessary
Never fast to the point where you go lightheaded or actually faint. If you get to this stage, eat a slice of bread or a biscuit to bring your blood sugar levels up and drink a sports drink that contains electrolytes.

You might feel lethargic for the first couple of days – do not give up because this will pass. Just allow yourself that time to relax and don't do anything strenuous.

Never do a liquid fast for any more than three consecutive days.

In the next chapter, we are going to take a look at what you can and shouldn't eat on a detox diet. I will also be giving you a few ideas for water recipes as well.

Chapter 3:

What You Should and Shouldn't Consume on a Detox Cleanse

The whole idea of a detox cleanse is to cut out the rubbish, the foods and drinks that contributing to that buildup of toxins in your body. Now, it can be a little confusing when you start a detox cleanse diet, knowing what you can and can't eat. So, the following lists should help to clear up any confusion you may have.

Foods to Eat

Fruits:

- Any fruit, fresh or frozen
- Fruit juices – must be natural and unsweetened – if in doubt, make your own
- Unsweetened dried fruit in small amounts – raisins, cranberries, goji berries, etc.

Vegetables:

- Broccoli
- Cauliflower
- Spinach
- Kale
- Beet greens

- Collard greens

- Onions

- Broccoli sprouts

- Garlic

- Beets

- Artichokes

- Swiss chard

- Kelp

- Nori

- Wakame

- Tomatoes

- Bell peppers

- Egg plants

- Potatoes (depending on the type of detox you are on)

- Avoid corn, as it is highly acid forming

Grains/Starches:

- Brown rice

- Quinoa

- Millet

- Buckwheat

- Wild rice

- Amaranth

- Oats

Go for whole grains where possible but you can use products made from the above, such as bread, buckwheat noodles, rice crackers, or brown rice pasta

Beans/Legumes:

- Adzuki
- Lima
- Kidney
- Green
- Black-eyed peas
- Lentils
- Split peas – green or yellow

Nuts/Seeds:

- Cashews
- Walnuts
- Almonds
- Sunflower seeds
- Sesame seeds
- Pumpkin seeds
- Chia seeds
- Hemp nuts
- Hemp seeds
- Young coconut
- Nut butters made with any of the above
- Tahini

Avoid peanuts or peanut butters and go for nuts and seeds that are unsalted and raw

Oils:

- Olive oil – cold-pressed, extra virgin is best
- Flax oil
- Hemp oil
- Almond oil
- Chia oil
- Avocado oil
- Coconut oil

You can consume safflower, sunflower, and sesame oils in small amounts

Foods to Avoid

Dairy/Eggs:

- Eggs in all formats
- Cheese
- Milk
- Sour cream
- Cottage cheese
- Kefir
- Yogurt, including frozen

Wheat:

- Butter
- Ice cream

Any product that contains wheat in any format, including bread or pasta, unless made with approved ingredients

Sweeteners:

- Sugar – refined, white, brown, castor, etc.
- HFCS – High Fructose Corn Syrup
- Cane juice
- Any artificial sweetener
- Any liquid sweetener

If you must use sweetener of any kind, use a little natural honey

Gluten:

- Wheat
- Rye
- Barley
- Spelt
- Kamut
- Triticale
- Bran
- Couscous
- Farina

Soy Products:

- Milk
- Tofu
- Yogurt
- Sauce
- Protein powder
- Tempeh
- Caffeine:

- Coffee

- Tea

- Soft drinks

You can drink decaffeinated coffee and green tea

Detox Waters

If you find yourself unable to face drinking liters of plain water every day, fear not. There are plenty of ways to spice it up a bit and give it a better taste in ways that can speed up weight loss, and cleanse you much quicker. Give some of these a shot and see how much fun it can be to drink water:

Slim-Down

This is amazingly beneficial water, helping to flush toxins out of the body and fat as well. Cucumbers are natural diuretics, which stop the water retention, and citrus fruits help to flush toxins and burn fat:

- ½ gallon spring water

- ½ a medium grapefruit

- ½ a cucumber

- ½ a lemon

- ½ a lime

- Mint leaves

Slice all the fruit and the cucumber up and add it all to the water in a large jug. Add the mint leaves and refrigerate for a couple of hours before drinking. Aim for at least ½ a gallon per day.

Fruity Detox

As well as tasting fantastic in the summer months, the fruit in this contains vitamin A and vitamin E, which both aid the flushing of free radicals and toxins. Strawberries are excellent for anti-aging and help the skin to stay smooth and youthful looking as well as helping to fight off carcinogens.

- 2 liters spring water
- 2 large strawberries
- Two small to medium kiwis

Chop the fruit and add to the water. Refrigerate for a couple of hours before use and drink at least 2 liters daily. Increase the fruit to taste

Day Spa Apple Cinnamon

This wonderful water contains absolutely no calories, making it marvelous for slimming and for flushing out the toxins. And, it can help to boost your metabolism, thus speeding up the weight loss.

- 2 liters spring water
- 1 apple
- 2 or 3 cinnamon sticks

Slice the apple thinly and place it into a gallon pitcher with the cinnamon. Fill up the jug halfway with ice and then add the water. Leave it in the fridge for about an hour before serving. You can fill this jug up three or four times without changing the apple or cinnamon and you can increase the fruit or cinnamon if you want a stronger taste

New Year Detox

This is a great water to drink any time of the year, not just at New Year. It's a great tasting water to help boost your metabolism, burn off fate and get rid of the toxins in your body.

- 1 gallon spring water
- Handful of raspberries
- 1 grapefruit
- 1 cucumber

- 1 pear
- Couple of sprigs of mint

Slice the grapefruit, pear, and cucumber and add to the water with the raspberries and mint. Refrigerate for a couple of hours before drinking. For a zestier taste, add limes, lemons, cranberries and blueberries as well

Strawberry Vitamin

Strawberry infused water not only flushes toxins out, it also helps to keep your skin looking youthful as well as being full of anti-inflammatory properties and vitamins.

- 2 liters spring water
- 1 cup strawberries
- 2 cups watermelon
- 2 sprigs fresh rosemary
- Dash of coarse sea salt

Cube the watermelon and place in a large jug. Chop the strawberries in half and mix together with the rosemary. Add to the jug and pour water over. Stir, add the salt, and refrigerate for 2 hours. Stir again before drinking

Fat Burner

This is wonderful detox water that flushes out the toxins, helps you to burn fat, and drop those pounds as well. It's full of fiber, and the cinnamon helps to slow down your appetite.

- 12 oz. spring water
- 2 tbsp. apple cider vinegar
- 1 tbsp. fresh lemon juice
- 1 tsp ground cinnamon
- Half a medium apple

Put all the ingredients, except the apple, into the blender for 10 seconds. Slice the apple, add to the drink, and enjoy

Cucumber Lemon Detox

Lemon is an excellent cleanser and helps to boost the immune system while cucumber is a diuretic that helps you to keep hydrated and has anti-inflammatory properties. The mint is good for digestion and helps to sweeten the water.

- 8 cups spring water
- 1 medium cucumber
- 1 lemon
- 10 mint leaves

Cut the cucumber and lemon into wedges or slice it – your choice. Add to the water with the mint and leave in the fridge overnight before drinking

Aloe

We all know what aloe Vera is but how many of us realize what the benefits of it are? It is excellent for aiding digestion and circulation as well as getting rid of fatigue.

- 1 cup water
- 2 tbsp. fresh lemon juice
- 2 tbsp. aloe gel

To get the gel, split an aloe leaf down the center and scoop the gel out. Add to the other ingredients in the blender and blend for about 1 minute before drinking.

Lemon Ginger

Ginger is one of the best natural pain relievers there is. Adding it to the cleansing properties of lemon gives you a great water to start every day with as it works to flush toxins all day long.

- 12 oz. water

- ½" chunk of ginger root

- ½ lemon juiced

Add the lemon juice to the water and grate the ginger in. Stir well and drink straightaway. Make sure your water is at room temperature

Detox Smoothies and Juices

As well as waters, you also have the option or making raw fruit and vegetable juices and smoothies, if you fancy something a little more filling. Try the following:

Matcha Mango Pineapple Smoothie Ingredients

- 1 ¼ cups of Matcha Matsu green tea

- 1 scoop of protein powder

- 1 cup of fresh or frozen (defrosted) mango chunks

- 1 tbsp. 100% pineapple juice

- 1 cup fresh or frozen (defrosted) pineapple chunks

- ½ - 1 cup of water

- Honey to taste

Add all the ingredients into the blender and blend until smooth. The amount of water you use depends on how thick you want your smoothie to be.

Cranberry, Kale and Pomegranate Detox Juice Ingredients

- 4-6 kale leaves, large ones

- 1 cup of pomegranate arils – from a large pomegranate

- cup fresh or frozen (defrosted) cranberries

- 1 pear, cored

- About an inch of fresh ginger, peeled

- 6-12 mint leaves – optional
- Stevia to taste

Put the ingredients, one at a time, into the juicer, leaving the pomegranate seeds until last. Strain if you want to and serve straightaway

Detox Vegetable Juice Ingredients

- 1 or 2 large red peppers, deseeds ad sliced up
- 4 sliced tomatoes
- 3 carrots, cleaned, peeled and sliced
- 2 heads of romaine lettuce
- 1 celery bunch
- A large handful of cilantro
- 1 cucumber, peeled and chopped
- 2 peeled lemons
- About an inch of fresh ginger

Juice everything together and give it a good stir. This will make around 3 pints but you can refrigerate for up to 48 hours – don't forget to give it a good stir before serving.

Grapefruit-Cado Sunrise Smoothie Ingredients

- ½ fresh avocado
- ½ cup orange juice, fresh squeezed
- 1 up grapefruit juice, fresh squeezed
- 1 cup frozen strawberries
- ¾ cup frozen banana slices
- ¼ cup ice
- 1 tsp maple syrup to taste, optional

Blend all the ingredients together until smooth and serve. You can substitute fresh squeezed juice for 100% natural juices but using fresh fruit is better

Orange, Apple Carrot, Celery and Lime Juice Ingredients

- 2 apples, quartered
- 2 cleaned carrots, chopped
- 1 celery stalk. Chopped
- 4-5 limes

Juice everything together until you have the desired consistency and serve over ice. You can add crushed ice into the blender if you want

Blueberry Fruit Smoothie Ingredients

- ½ cup frozen blueberries
- ¼ cup cranberry juice, unsweetened
- ½ bananas

Blend the entire ingredient together until smooth and serve immediately

Veggie Pizza Juice Ingredients

- 4-5 Roma tomatoes
- 2 sweet bell peppers, 1 yellow, 1 orange
- 1/3 yellow onion
- A bunch of kale
- 1 peeled garlic clove
- 10-15 basil leaves
- Handful of raw cashew pieces

First, juice all of the ingredients, leaving out the cashew pieces. Then pour the juice into a blender, add the cashews and blend

Carrot and Beet Smoothie Ingredients

- 1 peeled carrot, sliced

- 1 peeled beet, sliced

- ½ cup grapes, red

- 1 peeled clementine, broken into segments

- A slice of peeled ginger

- ½ cup green tea

Put the carrot and beet slices into a steamer and cook gently for about 10-15 minutes, or until tender. Leave these to cool off. Now add all of the ingredients to the blender and blend until smooth

Detox Meals

You do not need to starve yourself on a detox diet, far from it so below, I have given you just three recipes that you can eat while detoxing. These are just to give you a basis to start from and a few ideas.

Breakfast

Blueberry-Coconut Bakes Oatmeal Ingredients
OATMEAL

- 1 ½ cups steel cut oats

- ½ tsp ground ginger

- ½ tsp sea salt, fine

- 1 tsp baking powder

- 4 cups vanilla almond milk, unsweetened

- 2 cups light coconut milk, unsweetened

- 1 ½ cups fresh blueberries

- ¼ cup dried unsweetened blueberries

- ¼ cup coconut flak, unsweetened

- Natural sweetener to taste

BLUEBERRY SAUCE

- 2 cups blueberries, fresh or frozen

OPTIONAL TOPPINGS

- Coconut flake
- Toasted nuts
- Extra blueberries, dried or fresh
- Whipped cream
- Coconut milk

Preparation OATMEAL

1. Preheat the oven to 350° F and put the oven rack in the center
2. Coat a baking dish 13 x 9 x 2 inch lightly with cooking spray
3. Mix all of the oatmeal ingredients together, adding the coconut and blueberries last
4. Sweeten to taste and bake for approximately 1 hour
5. When the time is out, take the oatmeal out of the over, although it won't look cooked. Leave it to cool and then refrigerate overnight to thicken up

BLUEBERRY SAUCE

1. Add a splash of water to the blueberries and heat over a medium high heat
2. When they start to sizzle, reduce the heat and cook for 5 minutes, or until they turn to a sauce-like consistency
3. Mash them against the side of the pan
4. Serve the oatmeal with a little coconut or almond milk and the blueberry sauce

5   Use any of the additional toppings if you want but don't overdo it

Lunch

Baked Sweet Potato and Greens Ingredients

- 2 sweet potatoes, pricked
- 1 tbsp. extra virgin olive oil
- 1 small onion, sliced thinly
- 1 bunch Swiss chard, stemmed and chopped
- Coarse salt
- 1 avocado pitted and sliced
- Cayenne pepper
- Lemon

Preparation

1   Preheat the oven to 400° F

2   Bake the potatoes for about 45 minutes, or until tender

3   Heat the oil in skillet and cook the onion until tender, around 6 minutes

4   Add the chard, stirring, and cook until it is bright green and has wilted, around 5 minutes

5   Season with the salt

6   Split the potatoes and top each one off with the greens and half the avocado

7   Season with salt, cayenne and a squeeze of lemon

Dinner

Chicken, Vegetable, Avocado and Rice Bowls Ingredients

CHICKEN

- 1 lb. chicken breast, boneless and skinless (if using skewers, cube it, if not, leave it whole)
- ¼ cup olive oil
- 4 garlic cloves, minced
- ½ tsp onion powder
- ½ tsp pepper
- ½ tsp cayenne
- ½ tsp smoked paprika
- ¼ cup chopped fresh parsley or 1 tbsp. dried
- ¼ cup chopped fresh basil or 1 tbsp. dried

RICE AND VEGETABLES

- 1 ½ cups rice, Basmati or jasmine
- 3 cups water
- 2 red peppers, quartered
- 1 zucchini, cut into ¼ inch rounds
- 1 tbsp. olive oil
- Salt and pepper to taste
- 2 avocadoes, pitted, peeled and mashed thoroughly
- Juice from 1 lemon
- ½ cup chopped fresh parsley
- 1 clove grated garlic
- 1 pint of halved grape or cherry tomatoes

- ¼ cup toasted walnuts

- ½ cup crumbled blue cheese – optional

Preparation

1   If you are using bamboo skewers, soak them for 30 minutes before you start grilling to stop them from charring

2   In a bowl, mix the garlic, olive oil, onion powder, paprika, cayenne, basil and parsley. Add in the chicken and toss to coat

3   Cover the bowl and refrigerate while you are making the rice

4   To make the rice, bring the water to a low boil and then drop the rice in. Stir it well, cover and reduce the heat as low as possible

5   Cook for 10 minutes, turn off the heat and leave the rice for a farther 20 minutes, covered – do not uncover at all, not even to take a look

6   After the 20 minutes is up, remove the lid and use a fork to fluff up the rice

7   Reheat the grill to medium high

8   Put the pepper and zucchini in a large Ziploc bag

9   Add a pinch of salt and pepper and 1 tbsp. of olive oil 10 Seal the bag and shake to coat the vegetables
11 Remove the chicken form the refrigerator

12 Either skewer it or leave it whole and cop it after grilling

13 Grill for about 3-4 minutes either side, turning it a couple of times until thoroughly cooked and with light char marks across it

14 At the same time, grill the zucchini, about 4 minutes either side and the peppers for 5 minutes 15 Remove the food from the grill and leave for 5 minutes to cool down

16 Slice the peppers into strips and cut whole chicken breast into

cubes (if you are not skewering it)

17 Put the avocado mash into a bowl, add the garlic, parsley, salt, pepper and lemon juice to taste, stirring well

18 Divide the rice over 4 serving bowls

19 Top each one with chicken, pepper and zucchini (or a couple of skewers)

20 Add a large spoon of the avocado mix and top off with tomatoes and walnuts, sprinkling blue cheese over if you want to

21 Serve immediately

15 Detox Salads

Salads do not need to be boring! Most people turn their noses up at salad because they think only of the basics, like lettuce, tomato and cucumber. While these do make a very nice salad, there are tons of other ingredients that you can add. Most salads have a detox effect on the body but the ones I am going to tell you about are especially detoxifying and will help to clean your system out a bit.

A detox salad is nothing more than a bunch of ingredients that all have a detox effect. A lot of the time, we chop these ingredients up finely, to allow for easier chewing and digestion. A lot of these ingredients are high in fiber, which helps your digestive system to work properly, and some are designed to clean the kidneys and the liver. Yet others will help to stock up your body with the nutrients and vitamins it so badly needs. Each of these salads is different, and each has its own effect on your body. I am not giving you exact recipes here, just the ingredients – use them in the quantities that you want!

1. Rainbow Salad and Roast Squash

This is a very pretty salad but, aside from that, it is highly beneficial to the body. The roast squash blends very well

with the rest of the ingredients to provide a filling and satisfying salad that will keep you full for some time. Simple slice and deseed a small squash, leaving the skin on. Season with salt and pepper before roasting. Steam some broccoli florets. Mix tender greens, diced red onion, sliced red cabbage, radishes and pumpkin seeds together in a bowl. Serve topped with the roast squash and broccoli and the (healthy) dressing of your choice for a salad that is full of fiber.

2. Simple Detox Salad

While this might look like a basic salad, it is much more. The ingredients will be working hard to deliver fiber, nutrients and vitamins, as well as healthy fats, antioxidants and potassium, all designed to help the body rid itself of toxins. Simply take a bunch of kale that has been de-stemmed and chopped up and add it to red cabbage, carrots, black beans, mushrooms, roasted beets, red peppers, sunflower seeds and roasted Brussels sprouts. Top off with half an avocado.

3. Winter Detox Salad

So many people think salads are just for warmer weather and detoxing is only for the spring months but this salad is perfect for a cold gray winter's day. In the winter, our bodies tend to retain more of what we eat and we need to get that digestive system moving so you are not building up a body full of toxins. That is exactly what this salad is for. Chop up a couple of medium sized rutabaga heads and add grated carrot, pomegranate seed, pine nuts and pink peppers. Make a dressing from olive oil, fresh lemon juice and pink Himalayan salt and toss the salad in it.

4. Quinoa, Almond and Apple

You do not need to stick to vegetables for a perfect salad. Instead, fruits, nuts and grains can do just as good a job of cleansing your body. Quinoa is filling; apple is full of nutrients, as well as being a superfood as are the almonds. Cook the quinoa and allow to cool. Mix with toasted chopped almonds, diced apple, cranberries and scallions for a tasty healthy salad.

5. Cauliflower and Broccoli Detox Salad

Both of these vegetables are members of the cruciferous family and, while they taste completely different, the benefits they give you are somewhat similar. Both contain heaps of vitamins and nutrients and, with the addition of the carrots and the sunflower seeds give you a complete body cleanse. Mix steamed broccoli and cauliflower florets with shredded carrot, sunflower seeds, currants, raisins and fresh parsley. Season with a little salt and lots of pepper, drizzle lemon juice over and, if you can get them, or indeed want them, add a sprinkling of kelp granules.

6. Shredded Vegetable Salad

The idea behind shredding everything is that it makes it easier to chew and is easier on the digestive system too. You can make up a big bath of this on and eat it for a few days but do drizzle lemon juice and olive oil over it to preserve it for longer. Use your food processor to shred carrots, and then chop the cauliflower, kale, broccoli and parsley into very small chunks. Toss together with sunflower seeds and raisins and dress with lemon juice and olive oil.

7. Gluten-Free

Not everyone can eat foods that contain gluten so you need to choose detox foods that keep you to your gluten-free lifestyle. Most of the salads on this list are actually gluten-free but sometimes there is the odd ingredient that contains it. And, because this salad contains no animal byproducts, it's also a great one for vegans. Process broccoli and cauliflower into very small pieces and do the same with a carrot. Mix together in a bowl and add in fine chopped kale, sunflower seeds, chopped parsley, sliced almonds, currants and blueberries. Mix lemon juice, mild vinegar and maple syrup for a dressing and add kelp powder if you want to.

8. Kale Salad

All too often, we are told we must eat more kale but there are only so many ways you can eat it. As well as mixing it in green smoothies, you can also add it to this tasty salad. The addition of cucumber helps with hydration as well as balancing the kale taste out as well. Avocado gives you a healthy dose of the good fats, making it a fully cleansing super-salad. Mix sliced kale and chopped scallions with shelled edamame and diced cucumber. Dice the avocado and toss it in lemon juice before adding it to the salad. Make a dressing from olive oil, lemon zest, mirin, cayenne, ginger and salt and drizzle over the salad. Toss well and top off with pinenuts or sunflower seeds.

9. Asparagus and Tomato Salad

One common misconception about salads is that they have to have lots of different ingredients to actually be classed as a salad. Some of the best salads have only a couple of ingredients that go well together, Asparagus and tomatoes are two of those foods, both providing nutritious and cleansing benefits to the body. Thinly slice a bunch of raw asparagus and mix it with halved cherry tomatoes. Make a dressing from lemon juice, vinegar, salt and pepper and toss the asparagus and tomatoes in it. You can add a sprinkling of shaved parmesan cheese as well if you want it.

10. Roasted Beets and Pumpkin Seeds

Roasted beets are a fantastic detox food – but only if you use raw beets that you cook, NOT pickled ones. The addition of pumpkin seeds and greens completes this bountiful salad full of fiber and nutrition, as well as antioxidants. Cook and cool the beetroots or buy them ready cooked. Cut into cubes. Put mesclun greens, or whichever you prefer, into a bowl and top with the beet cubes and pumpkin seeds. You can add crumbled goats cheese if you want but it isn't a highly detoxifying food. Drizzle a dressing made from olive oil and balsamic vinegar over the salad and enjoy – both you and your liver!

11. Everyday Detox Salad

You don't have to make detoxing a one-off thing; you can give your body exactly what it needs every single day. This salad combines miso and carrot for a tasty dressing that will make you crave this over and over again. The salad is based on that healthy superfood spinach with cucumbers and tomatoes providing a flavorsome, nutrient dense salad. To make this salad, chop up a spinach, red onion, cherry tomatoes, cucumbers, and cilantro and mix it all together in a bowl. Make the dressing from chopped carrots and shallots, grated ginger, white miso paste rice vinegar. Sesame oil, water and vegetable or olive oil – just mix it all up and toss your salad in it.

12. The Happy Salad

The name really does say it all here – your body will be over the moon if you give it this salad on a regular basis and you will be giving it exactly what it needs in terms of nutrition. The ingredients in this salad ensure that you will have more energy and your elimination system will be more regular, making you feel good in body and mind. Chop carrots, green cabbage, green onions and steamed broccoli. Make a dressing from maple syrup, lemon zest, minced garlic, minced or grated ginger and add a little salt and pepper. Toss your salad in it and sprinkle a few sunflower seed kernels over the top – as many as you want really.

13. The Day after Detox Salad

We all go through days and nights of heavy celebration – weddings, birthdays, holiday season, etc. – and this salad is designed for the day after a bag over indulgence. It is standard as far as detox salads go but it does have one ingredient that is scientifically proven to provide your intestines with healthy flora, thus helping your digestive system to get moving and your elimination system to work properly. You need some roughly chopped carrots. Steamed broccoli chopped up. Grape tomatoes, sunflower seeds, all mixed and tossed in a dressing made from grapeseed oil, apple cider vinegar, nutritional yeast, lemon juice, salt and pepper. Leave it chilling in the refrigerator for about 30 minutes before you eat it.

14. Citrus, Seeds and Greens Salad

Citrus fruits are known for their naturally cleansing properties, which makes them the perfect addition to any detox diet. Every ingredient in this salad will hit your body with bolts of goodness and nutrition. The contrast between the tart citrus, the bitter greens and the crunchy nuts will be an assault on your taste buds, one that you will keep going back for time and time again. And if you really don't like the taste of greens then this is the perfect salad for you – you get a healthy serving of them with their taste disguised almost completely by the citrus.

You need a big bunch of greens – lettuce, spinach, arugula, rocket, etc. – a grapefruit, an orange, a lemon, sunflower seeds and pumpkin seeds. Mix it altogether, drizzle a little olive oil over the top, season with salt and pepper and enjoy.

15. Detox Slaw

This is a slaw that has delusions of being a salad or it could be a salad that thinks it might be a slaw. Whichever way it is, you can be sure you are getting a healthy dose of vegetables, especially cabbage. Cabbage is a wonderful superfood and you really should eat more of it. You don't need to shred this as much as you would a normal slaw ether so your teeth can get a bit of exercise too.

You will need red and green cabbage, carrots, fresh ginger, shelled edamame, radishes, water, salt, garlic, sherry vinegar, a shallot, olive oil and a lime. Shred the vegetables and mix them together. Then toss them in a dressing made from radish, carrot, miso paste, water, vinegar, ginger, lime and olive oil. Add a bit of garlic for good measure.

18 Teas for a Daily Detox Cleanse

Tea drinking may be something of a British custom but anyone can enjoy a daily cup of cleansing tea. Detox teas are soothing, and if you drink a different one off this list every day, you will be getting the full range of cleansing and detoxifying effects. These teas are idea for filling you with healthy nutrients and antioxidants at a cost that any pocket can afford. All of these teas can be bought from health stores, pharmacies or supermarkets. Or, if you choose, you can make your own.

1. Burdock Root Tea

Burdock is one of the little-know herbs that is full of detoxifying properties. As well as helping to purify the blood, it can strengthen your immune system. It is perfect for the liver and for the digestive system, which are the two main detox paths that the human body has. If your liver is functioning well, you will have less toxins in your blood and if your digestive system is working to keep you regular, the toxins won't have a chance to build up.

2. Cayenne Pepper Tea

It is only recently that cayenne pepper has become popular for its health benefits and more people are starting to use it to spice up their meals. However, it can also be brewed up as a tea and, in this format, it will give you a healthy dose of energy while cleansing your body. If you don't like it too spicy, add a slice of lemon. This will take the edge off the spice, cleanse the palate and help your digestive system get moving.

3. Chicory Tea

Chicory tea is fantastic for detoxing the body and it can also help to give your metabolism a huge boost, giving you a double dose of goodness. Chicory is good for getting the digestive juices revved up before you eat, making it easier to digest your food. If you choose to make this yourself use dried chicory as it contains more taste, more of the essence and plenty of vitamins.

4. Cilantro Tea

Most people add cilantro to their food to provide a strong taste but you can make a perfectly good detox tea from it as well. Cilantro is fast becoming one of the most popular herbs that helps enormously with the digestive system. It can help your body to better process foods by breaking them down more efficiently and making use of more of the nutrients, before it effective eliminates what isn't needed.

5. Dandelion tea

Dandelions are always seen as a bad weed in the garden but they are one of the most purifying "weeds" ever grown. Scientific research has shown that dandelion increases the levels of a particular enzyme that is known for being a detoxifying enzyme. They have also been known to remove toxins that may cause cancer from the body as well, making it extremely worthwhile to drink.

6. Fenugreek Tea

Fenugreek is known for helping with the digestion and can be very helpful whenever you feel as though your digestive system has sowed right down. For some people who constantly feel bloated or suffer with indigestion, this can be a daily drink. Other might find it beneficial to drink once a week. There are also some other benefits to drinking fenugreek tea; it can lower your blood pressure and help to reduce inflammation in the body.

7. Garlic Tea

Everyone should already know of the massive benefits that garlic provides and drinking it made into a tea is hugely cleansing. This is because it is full of vitamins and sulfur which is one of the most effective ingredients for detoxifying the body.

8. Ginger Tea

Ginger is another food that is excellent for cleansing the body and it tastes lovely brewed up as a tea. It is very gentle on your body, despite the tartness it has and that makes it perfect for daily use. Not only is it good at helping with detoxification, it can also be used as warming drink or as a pick-me-up and a boost to energy levels.

9. Green Tea

Green tea has amazing benefits and is one of the most widely written about teas. It has been scientifically proven that drinking one cup of green tea every day will improve your health no end. It is packed full of antioxidants that fight against free radicals and tons of other toxins and it has one other added benefit – the removal of all those toxins helps you to shed weight without even trying.

10. Guduchi Tea

You may not have heard of this herb but you should give it a go. It has long been used in many parts of the world for its restorative properties and it contains a long list of benefits. Those benefits include improving your skin, ridding the body of toxins and helping with the digestive system, amongst many others and this is all because it assist the organs to work the way they should do.

11. Gymnema Sylvestre Tea

This is a Chinese herb that has major effects on glucose. We all know that too much blood sugar can be extremely toxic and this tea helps to regulate that as well as helping your body to function properly. It can help with the liver and the digestive system so it is definitely one to try.

12. Manjistha Tea

The skin is the single largest organ of the human body and that makes it one of the biggest ways to remove toxins. If your skin is not getting the right nutrients and the support that it needs, it can't help in the detox process. Manjistha is a plant that is full of medicinal properties that work well when it is drunk. It is also an excellent choice for women who suffer with bad menstrual problems, because of the effect it has on helping to purify the blood.

13. Milk Thistle Tea

Milk thistle contains huge benefits for the liver, which is the focal point for most of the other organs in the body. This means that when your liver is functioning properly, neither are your other organs. Your liver should be the main focus of any detox plan you undertake and milk thistle is perfect for that. It is also good for the digestive system, thus doubling the detox effect.

14. Neem Tea

Neem is an herb that is highly popular in India and it can drunk as a tea to ward off loads of different diseases and conditions. It helps the liver to perform better and is full of minerals and vitamins that the body needs on a daily basis.

15. Red Clover Tea

Red clover is packed full of antioxidants which help the body to fight off free radicals that we consume with our food and breather in from our environment. Daily boosts of these antioxidants is vital to stop the free radicals from accumulating in the body. Without any defense mechanism in pace, those free radicals can cause all sorts of conditions that you really don't want.

16. Triphala Tea

Triphala is used to stimulate the bowels and is often used as a way of treating constipation. The toxins that build up in your body have to be eliminated somehow and if the colon and bowels are not working like they should, the toxins will simply build up and end up being reintroduced back into your body. Triphala tea, drunk daily, or even a couple of times a week will stop this from happening.

17. Turmeric Tea

Many people use turmeric as a way of spicing up a meal but it can also be made into a tea very easily. Turmeric is one of the most potent natural anti-inflammatories that can help with all sorts of problems caused by inflammation. It can also help the liver and kick start the gallbladder into producing bile, which is needed to help break the toxins down and get them out of your body. Taken on a daily basis, turmeric is a great way to get your digestive system working optimally.

18. Wormwood Tea

Wormwood is an herb that helps the bile to get out of the liver and out of your body, which is useful to stop toxic buildups from stagnating in the body. Wormwood has a purging effect and is perfect as a daily tea to ensure that your body is making sufficient bile and that it is getting through your system, as it should.

10 Cleansing and Revitalizing Soups

Detox soups contain many of the best and healthiest ingredients there are and bring them altogether in one delicious pot. Mostly you will need to blend or puree the vegetables or very finely chop them for best results. Doing this makes it easier on your body to digest them and that means your body gets to absorb more of the nutrients. The best bit about these soups is that they all taste beautiful while giving you a good dose of detoxifying minerals and vitamins.

Hot and Sour Soup – Vegetarian

This soup uses apple cider vinegar to give it the sour taste. Apple cider vinegar is widely known for its qualities in helping to replenish digestive flora. Use a mixed mushroom pack or use shitake or reishi mushrooms, both known for having detoxifying properties.

Ingredients:

- 1 oz. mixed dried mushrooms
- 8 cups water
- 3 tbsp. sherry wine for cooking
- ¼ cup apple cider vinegar
- 2 tbsp. soy sauce
- 1 ½ tsp kosher salt
- 1 tbsp. grated ginger

- 1 lb. tofu, extra firm, cut into cubes of ½ inch

- 2 tbsp. cornstarch

- 2 lightly beaten eggs

- 6 trimmed and sliced scallions

- ¼ tsp white pepper

- Pure sesame oil for serving

Instructions:

- Put the mushrooms into a bowl containing 2 cups of boiling water. Cover and leave for at least 30 minutes to rehydrate

- Strain the mushrooms, retaining the water for the soup

- Slice them thinly

- Add the remaining 6 cups of water to the mushroom liquid in a soup pot and then add the mushrooms

- Bring to the boil and add the vinegar, sherry, salt, soy sauce, tofu and ginger. Turn the heat down and simmer for 10 minutes, uncovered

- Take about ¾ a cup from the broth and mix the cornstarch in until it has dissolved

- Pour back into the soup, stirring to ensure it is distributed – the soup should slightly thicken

- Keep stirring and pour the eggs into the soup

- Add the pepper and scallions and cook for another couple of minutes

- Serve with a drizzle of the sesame oil

Spicy Tender Green Soup

With celery as a base, you can't go wrong with this soup. Celery is a wonderfully cleansing vegetable that we really don't eat enough of but this soup makes it easy to get a real dose of vitamins and nutrients to help cleanse your body and fill you up with fiber.

Ingredients – serves 2

- 4 stalks celery
- 1 yellow onion
- 1 bell pepper – green
- 5 generous handfuls of spinach
- 2 cloves garlic
- ½ tsp cardamom
- ½ tsp ground ginger
- ½ tsp ground cumin
- 1 tsp ground mint
- 1 liter water
- Fresh ground black pepper and seas salt for seasoning
- Optional – coconut milk or cream

Instructions:

- Bring the water to a boil and add sea salt to taste
- Chop up the celery, pepper, onion and spinach and add them to the water
- Cover the pot and cook over a medium heat for about 15 minutes or until the vegetables have softened up
- Turn the heat off and add the whole garlic cloves.

- Blend the soup and serve with black pepper and cream or coconut milk if desired

Radish and Leek Soup

The humble radish gets nowhere near the respect it deserves but by adding it to this soup with leeks, you get a double nutritious punch. Potato gives the soup some texture and sea kelp finishes it off nicely. Radishes have a subtle taste when cooked if you do not use too many and are known as a cancer fighting food and a blood purifier.

Ingredients:

- ¾ lb. radishes, cut in half
- 3 Yukon potatoes, peeled and cut into cubes
- 2 whole trimmed leeks
- 32 oz. chicken broth
- 1-2 tsp sea kelp seasoning
- 2 tbsp. butter
- 1 cup milk, whole
- Salt and pepper for seasoning

Instructions:

- Separate the leek tops and slice them up the stalk. Wash the leaves well and set to one side
- Put the butter in a pot and turn the heat up. Add the radishes, potatoes and sea kelp seasoning
- Mix well and then add the chicken broth. Stand the leek leaves up in the pot and bring the soup to a boil before reducing the heat to a simmer
- Leave to simmer for 60 minutes or until the vegetables have

softened. Remove the leek tops and blend the soup in a blender

- Add the milk, blend again, serve with salt, and pepper to taste.

Lentil, Sweet Potato and Kale Stew

One of the best ways to get a detox soup or stew is to use foods together that are superfoods on their own. Lentils are great for keeping the digestive system on the move and the kale is just one of the best superfoods you could ever eat, being full of nutrients and antioxidants. The sweet potatoes add extra fiber and a broad range of nutrients.

Ingredients:

- 1 can diced tomatoes, low sodium variety
- 2 cups of chicken or vegetable broth, low sodium
- 1 cup dried green lentils
- 1 bell pepper, green or red, diced
- 1 tbsp. curry powder
- Pinch of cumin or garam masala (optional
- 3 cloves of garlic
- 1 bunch coarsely chopped kale
- 2 cups if water
- 1 small zucchini, diced (optional)

Instructions

- Sauté the onions in a little olive oil
- After 3 minutes, add the potatoes, curry powder and garlic
- Sauté for 5 minutes until all the vegetables are tender
- Add the tomatoes, broth, lentils and water
- Simmer for 45 minutes over a low heat or until the lentils

have gone tender

- Add the pepper and kale right at the end and cook for 10 more minutes
- Serve and enjoy

Healthy Detox Soup

When you have kale in your kitchen, you can add it to any soup to turn it into a detox soup. In this soup there are lots more vegetables that support the kale and provide a broad spectrum of minerals, vitamins and other nutrients. The citrus from the lemon provides a cleansing benefit and the pepper helps the body to absorb the nutrients from the rest of the vegetables

Ingredients:

- 2 medium leeks, halved, cleaned and chopped into small chunks
- 4 cloves garlic, crushed to a paste
- 1 serrano pepper, thinly sliced with half of the seeds taken out
- 4 carrots, cleaned and cut into chunks – leave the skins on
- 4 stalks celery, cut into chunks
- 3 small rutabagas, peeled and medium diced
- 3 small diced zucchini
- 8 cups water
- 3 Roma tomatoes, diced with the skin and the seeds
- 2 cups Pint beans
- 2 bunches thin sliced kale
- Sale and fresh cracked black pepper for seasoning
- Juice from ½ lemon

Instructions

- Heat up a large pot over a medium heat and then add the garlic, serrano pepper and leeks
- Sweat the vegetables on a low heat for 5 minutes, stirring regularly
- Add the rutabaga, celery and carrots and cook for a further 3 minutes
- Add the beans, water and tomatoes and simmer on a low heat for 30 minutes or more – the longer you leave it, the better the flavor
- About 15 minutes before you are due to serve it, add the zucchini and kale
- Cook for 5 minutes before stirring n the lemon juice
- Season with the salt and pepper and serve hot.

Potassium Balancing Soup

Potassium is a vital nutrient that many of us forget about. Luckily, if your levs are too low it is very easy to fix, simply by eating more foods that are rich in the nutrient. This soup is designed to boost your potassium intake in more than one way. The kale has 329 milligrams of potassium per cup and carrots are not much less than that. The avocado is optional but it too contains a whole load of potassium, more than there is in one banana, as well as containing a whole bunch of other nutrients and healthy fats.

Ingredients:

- 3 large or 4 medium zucchini
- 4-6 large kale leaves
- 3-4 onions – green or spring
- 2 carrots

- 3 stalks of celery – if you are on a very low sodium diet leave these out.

- 1 lb. fresh green beans

- Bunch of fresh parsley

- Handful of cilantro (coriander)

- 3 tomatoes or a can of chopped tomatoes, low sodium variety

- 3 cloves of garlic

- 3 tbsp. tamari – omit if you are on a low sodium or a migraine diet

- 2 tbsp. seaweed flakes or use 1-2 sheets of nori, toasted and crumbled up – not if you are on a migraine diet

- 2 tbsp. amaranth or teff seeds – optional

- 1 sliced avocado

Instructions

- Wash the vegetables and put ach one through your food processor, chopping finely, one vegetable type at a time – make sure you leave the stems on the kale as this is where the potassium is

- Keep a bit of parsley back for garnishing

- Add each chopped vegetable to a heavy stock pot

- When the last one is in, add 1 liter of filtered or spring water

- Add the tamari, seaweed and teff or amaranth seeds, stirring well

- Bring up to a gentle boil, reduce the heat, cover and simmer for 30 minutes before serving

Kale and Lentil Soup

While kale and lentils are the named vegetables in this soup, there are loads of other that are great for your detox plan. If you just ate kale on its own, your body would be getting a detox; add the lentils and you get extra fiber, boosting your digestive system. The addition of parsley, garlic and carrots makes this a truly cleansing and highly nutritional soup.

Ingredients

- 8 cups of vegetable broth
- 1 ½ cups rinsed red lentils
- 2 carrots, cleaned and chopped
- 2 diced onions
- 1 bunch of kale, de-stemmed and roughly chopped
- 1 clove of garlic
- ¼ tsp red pepper flakes – optional
- 1 tbsp. chopped parsley – chop first and then measure
- Zest from ½ a lemon

Instructions

- Put the vegetable broth into a large saucepan with the carrots, lentils, garlic, onions and kale
- Bring up to the boil and cook for about 15 or 20 minutes, until the lentils are tender
- Add the red pepper flakes if using, the zest and parley
- Stir well and serve hot

Broccoli and Pea Pot

You cannot go wrong if you eat broccoli and adding it to any dish turns that dish into a detox recipe. Each serving of this soup contains ¼ lb. of broccoli and the lentils provide a good boost of fiber as well as protein.

The rest of the ingredients simply reinforce this thick soup as perfect for detoxing.

Ingredients

- 1 tbsp. olive oil
- ¼ cup green onions, chopped
- 1 finely chopped shallot
- 1 lb. of broccoli florets
- 1 tbsp. fresh thyme leaves
- ¼ tsp salt
- ½ tsp ground black pepper
- 3 cups of vegetable broth – homemade is best if you have some
- ¾ cup peas, frozen and thawed out is fine
- ¾ cup cooked brown or green lentils
- 1-2 cups of fresh spinach, de-stemmed and cleaned, torn into small chunks

Instructions

- Heat up a little oil in a heavy pan until it is hot and then add the shallots and green onion
- Cook for about 3-5 minutes, stirring constantly
- Add in the broccoli, salt, pepper and thyme – sauté for about 5 minutes
- Add the broth and bring it up to the boil
- Add in the peas and the lentils and then cook for another 5-10 minutes, or until the vegetables have softened to tender
- Cool it slightly and then add the spinach

- Separating the soup into smaller batches, puree it in a blender until it is smooth and creamy

- Put back in the pot and heat on a low heat until hot

- Add salt and pepper to taste and serve hot

Detox Green Machine Soup

Spinach makes an appearance in this recipe. It is one of the most nutrition dense foods available but it should really be combined with other ingredients, otherwise your soup will end tasting only of spinach. Green beans, zucchini and celery provide a wonderful taste along with a whole bunch of vitamins and minerals why the garlic, parsley and basil ensure that you will keep returning to the pot time after time for more of this detoxifying soup.

Ingredients

- 1 lb. green beans, fresh or frozen and thawed will do well

- 8 sticks of celery

- 4 lb. zucchini

- 2 generous bunches of spinach

- 1 whole yellow onion

- 5 cloves of garlic

- 1 bunch of parsley

- 1 bunch of basil

Instructions

- Put the green beans, the celery and the zucchini into a steamer and steam for about 15 minutes, or until they are very soft. Do not boil as you will lose most of the nutrients

- Add the garlic, onion and spinach to the steamer. Cook for a further 5 minutes

- If you want your soup to be thick drain off the excess water.

- Add in the parley and the basil and puree the soup until it is smooth

- Add salt and pepper to taste and serve hot

Apple and Roast Butternut Squash Soup

Roasting up a butternut squash is time consuming but it is really worthwhile. Let's face it, store bought butternut soup does not cut the mustard when it comes to taste; you simply can't beat a homemade version. Combined with the humble superfood, the apple you create a soup that is wonderful for the body. And add in those spices and you have a truly cleansing soup.

Ingredients

- 2-3 lb. of butternut squash, cut into 1 inch cubes

- 4 large apple, sweet ones like a Honeycrisp or a Gala, cut into 1 inch cubes

- 4 stalks of celery, chopped into 2 inch pieces

- 8 oz. mushrooms, halved

- 1 large onion cut into quarters

- ¼ cup of olive oil, a good quality one

- 4 cups of chicken or vegetable broth, low sodium

- 1 cup apple juice

- 2 tsp salt plus a little extra for taste

- 1 tsp black pepper pus a bit extra for taste

- ½ tsp nutmeg

- 1 tsp cinnamon

- ½ tsp red pepper flakes – optional if you want a bit of an extra kick to the soup

- Pumpkin seeds for garnish – optional

Instructions

- Preheat the oven to 425° F or 220° C
- Mix the butternut squash cubes with the onion and about a eighth of a cup of good quality olive oil
- Star to coat the butternut thoroughly
- Put the onion and butternut into a large roasting tin, together with the oil and back for about 30-40 minutes, or until the squash is tender to put a fork through
- Mix the apples with the mushrooms and the rest of the oil
- Put these into another roasting tin and bake until soft and fragrant, about 15-20 minutes
- Pour the broth into a large soup pan; add the apple juice and all of the roasted vegetables. Stir well
- Use an immersion blender to puree the vegetables and liquid in the pot. Alternatively, you can puree the vegetables in your blender first, along with the liquid; although you may need to do this isbatches.
- If the consistency is too thick, add a little more broth or water.
- Simmer over a low-medium heat until hot
- Season with the spices, stirring them in well to distribute
- Serve hot garnished with the pumpkin seeds or, if you prefer a little fresh parsley or thyme and a swirl of cream.

Chapter 4:

7 Steps to Detox Your Body From Sugar

You might not think of sugar as something that you need to detox from but there are a couple of factors that influence this – the first is that sugar is not natural and the second is that human beings have only really been eating sugar for a relatively short period of time. This should make you realize that it is something that should only be eaten in small quantities yet, much of what you eat has sugar in it. In fact, many of our foods are loaded with sugar and it isn't really your fault that you eat too much of it. Sugar is a highly addictive substance but there is something you can do – first, become consciously aware of how much sugar you are eating and second, do something about purging your body of the sugar and your cravings for it. The following seven steps are designed to help your body and mind detox from the sugar monster.

Step 1 – Wean yourself off gradually or go cold turkey – your choice

You are the only person that truly knows you so only you can decide whether to cut sugar from your life gradually or in one hit. To be fair, both ways can be very successful but only if they are applied to right personality. Some people will respond best to a gradual reduction, while others respond better to a complete change. If you are at all unsure which one is you, start by weaning yourself off it gradually and see how you go. However you do it, this process is going to take time – there is no quick way to condition yourself not to crave sugar and all things that are sweet and it is going to be a tough habit to break.

Step 2 – Do a Candida Cleanse

Candida is a nasty beast that feeds on the sugar you eat. When you stop feeding it, it causes you to create more. Candida is also responsible for making you want foods that are high in these tasty carbohydrates that are so bad for you, like pasta and bread. These foods all add to your weight and many of them contain sugar. There are lots of candida cleanses that you can do, each with its own method. One thing I can tell you – by cutting sugar out, you will NOT rid your body of candida so it is a good idea to do a cleanse anyway. This is the only way to kill off the fungus that cause you to crave the sugar in the first place.

Step 3 – Change to a natural form of sugar.

One part of a sugar detox is to get your body used to eating natural forms of sugar and not the manmade poison that has only been in our lives for a short time. Today's sugar has been highly refined and is engineered to make it cheap. There is a word of difference between organic raw honey and High Fructose Corn Syrup (HFCS) and the sooner you can flush out the refined sugar and move to natural forms, the better you will feel. Do be careful how much you eat though, because even natural sugars can give you a taste for the sweet stuff.

Step 4 – Exercise

Exercising more will hasten up the process of getting rid of these cravings. As well as keeping you busy and out of temptations way, exercise also provides a natural high. This high can easily replace the high that sugar gives you. It has been proven that, when you are looking to get rid of a toxic bad habit, the easiest way is to replace that with something else that gives you the same or better rewards. Exercise is a fantastic option because it occupies your mind, makes you feel better, gives you more energy and helps you to work off the pounds that the sugar has accumulated.

Step 5 – Check your food labels properly

Sugar is not always the easiest ingredient to find on a food label so what you need to do is learn all the different terms for the many different sugars in your foods. Quite apart from trying to spot the word "sugar", you should also look for anything that is syrup as these are usually made from sugar. Sweetener is another common word and you should also be looking for words like Maltose, Dextrose, lactose, Dextrin and Fructose. HCFS is another one you may see. The best thing to do is look at the total sugar content on the nutrition label if there is one. If sugar is listed, look through the ingredients to see which types. Some people just give up eating prepackaged and processed foods altogether because virtually all of them include some kind of sugar.

Step 6 – Don't make the mistake of switching sugar for an artificial sweetener

You can't get the best of your addiction to sugar by using artificial sweeteners because they are no better. Instead of making you feel better, all you are doing is switching sugar for a bunch of unknown chemicals that can actually cause worse health problems than sugar can. While many of these sweeteners may provide a sweet taste without actually being sugar, they are not very widely studies and what we do know about them is not good. If you must use one, go for something like Stevia or truvia because these are pure natural sugars that do not contain the chemicals.

Step 7 – Stay diligent

The single biggest setback you will face when you detox your body from sugar is a relapse. It may be just one soda or just one cookie but that can undo all the work you have done and set you back in your old ways. It never is just one, that is the nature of addiction and sugar is one of the most addictive substances in the food world. If you really feel that you are going to struggle, try cutting back for a month or so until you have more control over your cravings. If you do relapse, start again and do not get frustrated – that will just lead to you throwing the towel in.

Detox Desserts

Just so you don't think you are missing out altogether, there are some great desserts you can eat on a detox plan that use natural forms of sugar and taste fantastic.

Chia Pudding Ingredients

- 1 cup of regular milk, almond milk or coconut milk – unsweetened variety
- 1 tbsp. raw organic honey
- 2 tbsp. whole chia seeds

Instructions

- Put all the ingredients into a bowl and mix together thoroughly
- Leave to sit for about 2 minutes and then mix again so the mixture doesn't go lumpy
- If you end up using sweetened milk, do not use the honey as well

Detox Cookies Ingredients

- 3 bananas, very ripe
- ½ cup of unsweetened natural peanut butter or almond butter
- ½ cup high quality cocoa powder
- Handful of coarse sea salt for garnishing

Instructions

- Preheat the oven to 350° F
- Mash or puree the bananas until smooth – should be about 1

½ cups of puree

- Put the bananas in a large bowl and add the peanut or almond butter and the cocoa powder
- Use a fork to mix together until the ingredients are fully combined in a smooth consistency
- Grease or line a cookie sheet and put spoonful's of the mixture onto the sheet, leaving about an inch between them
- Sprinkle a little sea salt over the top
- Bake for about 8-15 minutes until the sheen on the cookies has gone
- Remove from the oven and leave to cool for a few minutes before transferring them to a wire rack

Detox Pancakes Ingredients

- 1/3 cup rolled oats
- 2 tbsp. ground flax seeds
- ½ tsp baking powder – sodium free
- ½ tsp cinnamon
- 2 packed cups of raw spinach
- 3 large egg whites
- ½ bananas – medium ripe
- ½ tsp vanilla extract

Instructions

- Heat up a non-stick pan and coat it with cooking spray
- Blend the oats and flour together in a blender or food processor
- Empty into a bowl and then add the cinnamon, baking powder and flax seeds, stirring to combine thoroughly

- Put the spinach, banana, egg white and vanilla into a blender and pulse until smooth

- Add to the dry ingredients and stir until they are fully incorporated

- Spoon the batter into the hot pan and form four medium pancakes

- Cook for about 4-6 minutes on each side or until the edges have started to go brown

- Serve with fresh fruit, yogurt and nuts **Green Tea and Ginger Banana Ice Cream – Vegan Ingredients**

- 1 frozen banana – to freeze a banana, peel it and break it in half, freeze in a freezer-safe container until you need it

- ¼ cup of strong green tea, cold

- ½ cup non-dairy milk, unsweetened – almond or coconut milk are good for this

- ¼ inch knob of peeled ginger

- Pinch of sea salt

- Stevia to taste – no other sweetener as this is a pure natural one

- Almond slivers and chocolate chips or nibs

Instructions

- Blend the milk, banana, green tea, salt and ginger until very smooth and whipped – it should have the texture of soft-serve ice cream

- Add in stevia to taste if you want it

- Add the toppings and enjoy or blend the toppings in and freeze for about an hour before consuming

Raw Chocolate Mousse – Vegan Ingredients

- ½ cup of raw cashews, unsalted variety
- ½ cup of unsweetened coconut milk
- 10 drops of stevia liquid OR ½ tsp powdered stevia
- ¼ tsp vanilla extract
- 1 avocado, ripe
- 1 ½ tbsp. raw cacao powder
- Pinch of sea salt

Instructions

- Blend the cashews with the milk, vanilla extract and stevia liquid – if you used powder leave it out of this step
- When blended, add in the salt, cacao and avocado along with the powdered stevia if necessary.
- Adjust the taste for salt and sweetness
- Serve chilled, garnished with a sprinkling of cacao powder or cinnamon

Chocolate Coconut Pudding Ingredients

- 1 1/3 cup of unsweetened coconut milk
- 1 cup of raw cacao powder
- 1 cup of raw organic honey or natural maple syrup
- 1 cup of dates, chopped and pitted – measure after chopping
- ¾ cup of dark chocolate chips or nibs
- 1 ½ avocadoes
- 1 banana
- 3 tbsp. coconut oil. Melted
- 1 tsp vanilla extract

- Pinch of cinnamon

Instructions

- Blend all of the ingredients together in a blender except for the chocolate chips
- When blended, stir the chocolate chips in
- Pour into bowls or glass chars and refrigerate for several hours

Healthy Detox Cookies Ingredients

- 1 ½ cups of raw walnuts, halved
- 1 cup (about 12) pitted dates
- ¼ tsp salt
- ½ tsp baking soda
- 1 tsp vanilla extract
- 1 flax egg – mix 1 tbsp. of chia or flax seeds with 3 tablespoons water and refrigerate for 15 minutes before use
- ½ cup dark chocolate chips – optional

Instructions

- Preheat the oven to 350° F
- Line a cookie or baking sheet with a silpat or lining paper
- Use an "s" blade in the food processor to blend the walnuts and dates together – it should form a crumbly texture
- Add the vanilla, baking soda, salt and the flax egg to the mix and blend until it's all smooth and a bit stickier than traditional cookie dough is
- Add the chocolate chips and pulse quickly just to combine them
- Put spoonful's of batter onto the lined sheet and flatten them

gently with your hands – wet your hands a little first so the dough doesn't stick

- Bake for 12 minutes or until the edges have started turning golden

- Remove from the oven and leave to cool for 10 minutes before turning them out onto a wire rack

Gluten-free Strawberry Squares Ingredients

For the filling

- 2 tbsp. cornstarch

- 2 tbsp. warm water

- 2 cups of strawberries diced finely

- ¼ cup maple syrup or raw organic honey

- ¼ tsp stevia or truvia powder For the base and topping
- 2 ¼ cups quick oats – not the whole rolled variety

- 1 tsp ground cinnamon

- 1 cup almond butter, natural peanut butter or sunflower seed butter – unsalted

- ¼ cup maple syrup or raw organic honey

- ¼ cup of apple butter – do not use applesauce as it is not the same

- 1 large egg, beaten

- ½ cup almonds, sliced

Directions

- Make the filling by combining the cornstarch and the warm water until the cornstarch has completely dissolved – there should be no clumps and it should be the consistency of milk. Set to one side and mix the strawberries with the honey/syrup and stevia in a pan over a medium heat

- Bring the pan to a boil and stir it well

- Remove from the heat and stir the cornstarch in, whisking it until it is smooth. Leave to cool

- Preheat the oven to 325° F and line an 8 x 8 baking tray with foil, enough so that it hangs over the edges of the tray

- Make the base and topping by combining the oats, apple butter, honey/syrup, cinnamon, almond butter and egg together. Combine until the oats have been moistened and all the ingredients are thoroughly mixed together.

- Press half of the mixture onto the baking tray and press it down firmly and evenly.

- Spread the strawberry mixture evenly over the top

- Add the almonds to the rest of the oat mixture and then crumble it over the top of the strawberry mixture

- Use a wooden spoon or spatula to press it down into the filling firmly – it must stick well

- Bake for about 25-30 minutes until the top has browned lightly

- Cool completely before you cut into squares

Blueberry Almond Muffins Ingredients for 6 muffins

- 1 cup of rice flour, brown

- ½ tsp baking soda

- 1 tsp baking powder

- ¼ tsp salt

- 7-8 large dates, dried

- ½ cup of unsweetened soy or almond milk

- 1 ½ tbsp. coarse ground flax seeds

- 1 tbsp. lemon juice

- ½ tsp lemon zest

- 1/3 cup applesauce, unsweetened

- ½ tsp vanilla extract

- ½ cup fresh blueberries

- ¼ cup toasted sliced almonds

Instructions

- Preheat the oven to 400° F

- Put liners into a 6 cup muffin pan

- Pulse the dates in a blender until they are finely chopped

- Add the applesauce and blend until the mixture is a smooth paste

- Combine the vanilla extract, milk, lemon zest and juice together and add the ground flax seed. Mix well and set to one side

- Whisk the rice flour, baking powder, baking soda and salt together and then add the wet ingredients. Mix until they are just combined

- Add in the almonds and blueberries and stir gently

- Spoon the batter into the 6 cups and bake in the center of the oven for 20-25 minutes – test with a toothpick. When it comes out clean, they are cooked

- Remove and allow to cool for 10 minutes or so before turning them out onto a wire rack

Cherry Garcia Ice Cream – Vegan and Detox Ingredients

- 2 cans full fat coconut milk – 15 oz. each
- 3 droppers of vanilla flavored stevia
- Pinch of salt
- 2 ½ tbsp. cornstarch
- 1 cup cherries, roughly chopped – frozen is fine
- 3 or 4 cherries extra for the base
- ½ cup chopped dark chocolate

Instructions

- Put all ingredients except for the cornstarch, stevia, salt and ¼ cup of the coconut milk together in a pan
- Bring up to a simmer
- Whisk the cornstarch with the rest of the milk until smooth and add to the saucepan
- Cook, stirring well, until the mixture has thickened up and coats the back of a wooden spoon
- Remove the pan from the heat and leave to cool to room temperature
- Put the mixture into a blender and add the remaining cherries; blend until the base is smooth and a light pink color
- Cover, chill for at least 4 hours, up to 24 hours
- Freeze in an ice cream maker as per the manufacturer's instructions and in the last couple of minutes, add in the cherry and chocolate mix. Serve straight away or put into the freezer.

Chapter 5:

How to Detox Your Body Every Day

A t the end of the day, we are all human beings. We all indulge at some time in our lives, admittedly some more than others and, in all honesty, there isn't any harm in the occasional glass of wine or a decadent dessert. It's when we do it all the time without taking preventative measures that the problems build up. There are things you can do every day that will help your body to detox, not just from the food you eat but from the daily onslaught of toxins, over which we have no control.

If you can't bear the thought of preparing for an intense detox, with a few changes to your diet and following the tips below, you can begin the process of detoxing your body every single day.

Drink Hot Lemon Water Every Morning

Drink a cup of hot or warm water with fresh lemon and cayenne every morning to kick-start your digestive system

Drink Cold Fresh-Pressed Juice

Preferably, on an empty stomach as your body will be able to better absorb all the nutrients. Try juicing kale, lemon, spinach, ginger and spirulina together!

Sip on a Detox Tea

Try a few cups throughout the day instead of water or coffee. Look for those that have licorice root, dandelion root, burdock and ginger in them

Use Apple Cider Vinegar

As often as you can, even add it to your juices and smoothies, or a teaspoon in your water. Apple cider vinegar alkalizes an acidic body and helps the liver to detox.

Eat Foods and Supplements That Detox

There are loads of different foods that you can choose from to help your liver and kidneys cleanse the body, including:

- Parsley
- Cilantro
- Dandelion root
- Licorice root
- Cayenne
- Turmeric
- Red pepper
- Garlic
- Lemon
- Lime
- Grapefruit
- Sea vegetables
- Beets
- Artichokes
- Cruciferous vegetables
- Spirulina
- Wheatgrass
- Chlorella
- Milk thistle

There are many more listed in this book that you can choose from as well

Eat Clean

More fiber in your diet to ensure your elimination process keeps on moving along smoothly. Limit the amount of fish that have a higher level of mercury such as:

- Swordfish
- Tuna
- Mackerel
- Shark
- Grouper
- Marlin

As a rule, the larger the fish, the more mercury it has. Avoid those processed foods, refined sugars, caffeine, alcohol and fruits or vegetables that are not organic.

Sweat it Out

As we discussed earlier, in order to get rid of toxins, you need to sweat. A sauna, light exercise, gardening, anything like that which makes you sweat will ultimately make your body cleaner and help to eliminate toxins. You can also try yoga.

Invert

Inverting has been categorically shown to stimulate the endocrine, lymphatic, nervous and cardiovascular systems because it reverses the flow of gravity. Some inversions you could have a go at are:

- A shoulder stand
- A headstand
- A hand stand
- Lying with your legs up against a wall

Jump

This is another activity that is good for stimulating circulation and the lymphatic system. Get a small portable trampoline and start adding jumping into your day.

Eliminate

Make sure you are getting plenty of fiber in your diet, as well as digestive enzymes, probiotics and go for a regular enema or colonic to keep your system clear.

Dry Body Brushing

Before you get in the shower or a bath, dry brush your entire body. Use lone strides of the brush towards the heart as this helps to get the lymphatic system activated and stimulates circulation, as well as helping to eliminate those toxins through the skin

Scrape Your Tongue

I bet you didn't expect to see that on the list! The tongue is the perfect place for bacteria to gather and any toxic debris that might have gathered overnight. Try and do this twice a day, while you are brushing your teeth and you will find that it helps enormously in releasing toxins from your body.

Hydrotherapy

Hydrotherapy sounds expensive and complicated but you can actually do this at home. Stand in your shower and turn the water on hot. After 30 seconds, turn it to cold and keep repeating this while you shower. The cold water helps to contract your blood vessels while the hot water causes them to dilate. By alternating hot and cold, your body's elimination process will be improved, inflammation decreases, waste is eliminated from body tissues and your circulation increased.

Detox Bath

This ideal to use after you have dry brushed your body. You should definitely have one of these baths one a week to help cleanse your system:

- 2 cups of Epsom salts
- 2 cups baking soda
- 1 tbsp. fresh ground ginger
- 4 drops each of geranium, juniper berry and eucalyptus essential oils

Add to your bath water and enjoy. Do make sure the essential oils are of the therapeutic grade, not the perfume grade as there is a vast difference between the two! The Epsom salts draw toxins out of the body through the skin, the baking soda alkalizes acid in the body and removes toxins while the ginger will heat up your temperature, helping you to perspire and we know that sweating is good for ridding us of toxins.

Make your House Healthy

Plants, like peace lilies, palms and ferns act as air filters, as well as looking nice. You should also make sure you change your air conditioning filters on a regular basis, do not use harsh household chemicals, have chlorine filters installed, get an air purifier and think about a reverse osmosis water system.

Detox Massage

One of the best forms of massage for inclusion in a detox plan is the manual lymphatic drainage massage. This form of massage uses gently strokes to stimulate the lymphatic system, encouraging it to eliminate any excess fluid, metabolic waste and bacteria. The effects of this kind of massage are many and includes benefits to the muscular system and the nervous system. It is a great addition to your detox plan as it encourages the fluid in the connective tissues to flow.

The lymphatic system is made up of lymph nodes, lymph vessels and organs. The lymph nodes are part of the defense system in the human body and they are responsible for removing microorganisms and other foreign bodies. They are a filter that keeps things like bacteria from getting into your blood stream and when the system becomes sluggish, all manner of things can get through.

Stimulating the lymphatic system through this kind of massage activates all of the system and it encourages cell regeneration and fluid circulation. Both of these are vital to proper detoxification, to speed up the healing process and to provide support to the immune system. Positive Health Online author, David Goddard ND, says:

"The lymphatic system has a vital role in the body by regulating the immune system, which protects the body against infection. It transports nutrients to cells and eliminates metabolic wastes, toxins and excess fluids from the body. Manual lymphatic drainage is also a very effective way of detoxing the body plus stimulating vital immune defenses. This is a powerful, deep cleansing treatment."

The Benefits of Manual Lymphatic Drainage

The real benefits of manual lymphatic drainage are:

- Clears congested areas, like puffy eyes, swollen ankles and swollen legs
- Promotes the healing of scar tissue, sprains, and torn ligaments
- Promotes post-operative healing
- Relieves swelling after plastic surgery
- Treats lymphedema and other conditions that may arise from venous insufficiency
- Promotes improvement in chronic conditions, like arthritis, sinusitis, acne and many other skin conditions

- Promotes deep relaxation

Do be careful to choose a properly trained therapist as this is a specific technique and must be done properly.

Simple Lymphatic Drainage – DIY

There is a way of helping your lymphatic system to drain and start moving again:

- Relax your fingers and place them gently on the sides of your neck, right underneath your ears
- Move the skin gently towards the back of your neck, using a downward motion
- Repeat this 10 times, moving your fingers gradually lower, away from your ears
- Now put your finger on either side of your neck at the tops of your shoulders
- Massage gently, moving the skin in towards the collarbone
- Repeat this 5 times.

Chapter 6:

7 Steps to Detox for Acne

I t is so easy to forget that all of our body is connected and that the lifestyle you lead has an impact on all of the different parts. By giving your body a good detox, you are cleansing it of all impurities and allowing all of your organs to work together in perfect harmony, as they should do. Your skin is the largest organ you have and it too will benefit greatly from cleansing, to allow all the impurities to come out and be replaced with minerals and nutrients needed for healthy and clear skin. The following steps are designed to help you prevent acne from breaking out:

Step 1 – Stop the toxins from flooding in

Part of the process of detoxing your body is to significantly reduce the amount of toxins that are going into it. Toxins come in many disguises and some may not be quite as obvious as others. Alcohol and tobacco smoke are obviously toxic but how many of you realize just how many different pesticides and herbicides you are taking in from fruits and vegetables you eat that are grown conventionally? What about the meat and dairy products you eat – many of those are full of antibiotics and growth hormones. Add to that the heavy metals that are taken into your body over time and your body will soon become blocked. One of the side effects of all these toxins is acne.

Step 2 – Start from the inside

Acne comes from within your skin so it makes sense for you to target the problem or prevent it from happening from the inside out. Acne isn't an indicator of what you may be doing in your life now, rather it indicates things that you have or haven't done over the last few years. Move the focus of your treatment to the inside of your body and you will see improvements within a short period of time. Keep the treatment up and the long term effects will be even more obvious:

- Drink lots of water – at least 2 liter per day. Dehydration can make acne worse.

- Do a colon cleanse. When waste builds up in your colon, it can manifest itself in unhealthy skin. Make sure you avoid caffeine and alcohol and eat foods that target the live

- Eat plenty of organic vegetables and fruits, as well as grass-fed organic meats and dairy products to limit your toxic consumption

- If you smoke, stop.

- Shower in filtered water to limit how much chlorine gets on your skin

Step 3 – Only use natural treatments for acne

Instead of using chemical laden treatments that can be harsh on the skin, use products that are natural and organic. Not only will these reduce the side effects of the chemical ones, they will also provide your skin with nourishment in the form of plants and herbs. Give your body what it needs, not chemical substances but all natural things.

Step 4 – Use a healing detox facemask

If you suffer from a severe acne problem, try using a healing detox facemask that is made with bentonite clay. This is known for its properties that draw toxins from the skin and is often used as part of the detox bath treatment. It will clear out your pores, removing impurities and any ingrained dirt, and if you use it on a weekly basis, it will help to keep your skin clean and glowing.

Step 5 – Watch the results

Some people expect to see instant results during a detox but, more often than not, things will get worse before they get better. This is because your body is pushing all those impurities out and, if you have never done an acne detox before, you might be a little worried at the initial results. Establishing good habits and allowing plenty of time to pass will provide you with the real results – better looking healthy skin that is free of impurities.

Step 6 – Fill in the gaps in your nutrition

Speak to your nutritionist to see if they think your acne could be caused by deficiencies in nutrients. You may not be getting enough of certain mineral or vitamin from what you are eating and this could be causing the problem. You may need to take supplements so make sure you go for the whole food vitamins, as these do not contain any synthetic materials

Step 7 – Keep it up

Getting on top of your acne and staying on top is not a quick sprint, instead it is more like a marathon. Yes, you may

well want your acne to disappear in a flash but there is no miracle cure and your body needs time to adjust to all the changes you are making. Trying to speed thing sup will just make things worse so take it easy, take your time and you will see the results you want.

Chapter 7:

7 Steps to Making Your Own Detox Body Wrap

The detox body wrap is fast becoming one of the more popular detox methods and it involves wrapping your body to help the toxins to draw out. There are a few ways to do this so you should choose the type of wrap that suits your current situation. Completing all of these steps should afford you a nice feeling of wellbeing and you will be at the start of your journey for better health.

Step 1 – Decide which type of wrap you want

There are a number of different wraps, each one having a different goal. Some are designed to draw the toxins out from the skin and use bentonite clay. There are wraps that just remove the impurities from your skin by doing a deep cleanse on the outer lay. And there are wraps that help you to work up a sweat and are designed with weight loss in mind as well. You will need to use a sauna unit for these to work so that the exceed water weight can be sweated out while your body is being infused with herbs and minerals. Choose the one that suits your requirements before you move on to the next step

Step 2 – Get everything together

Now you know which type of wrap you are going for, you will need to get everything together. You do need to get your bathroom ready for what you are about to do so cover all the surfaces with plastic wrap to keep them clean. This is easy than using sheets or towels because you won't need to wash the plastic wrap, just discard it and it will cover better. It will also avoid any staining as some of the clays and lotions you will need to use can stain worktops and fabrics

You will need elastic bandages to wrap yourself up in, the solution you have chosen for your body wrap and a sauna unit if necessary. Have plenty of clean towels to hand and a few spare as well

Step 3 – Prepare your space

Make sure you have plenty of room and that you will be able to move around without banging into things once you are wrapped. Move wastebaskets out of the way and clear off the countertops. This is meant to be a relaxing experience so the last thing you want to do is keep tripping over things.

Step 4 - Prepare your wrap

Follow the instructions on the detox solution you are using. Most of them involve soaking the bandage in the solution and then wrapping them around yourself. Do follow any specific instructions to the letter so that you don't miss anything out. You will likely only have enough of the solution to do this once so there is no room for mistakes and you don't want to run out before you have finished covering yourself.

Step 5 – Wrap up

Before you start, have a shower to make sure you are clean. If you feel it necessary, exfoliate your skin as well this may make the detox solution soak in a little better. Start wrapping from your feet and work your way up your body, leaving your arms until last – you may need a little help to do the last one. If you are using the sauna nit method, get in; if not, lay in the bathtub – an empty one – so that the solution does not stain anywhere else. Cover the bathtub with plastic wrap first and make sure the room is a comfortable temperature.

Step 6 – Relax your body and mind

It might seem hard to relax while you are wrapped up like a mummy but if you start with your mind, your body will follow. Think positive thoughts. Detoxing isn't just about the body; it is also about the mind and ridding it of toxic thoughts. Think of things that make you feel good or think about what you are doing and the results you are hoping to achieve.

Step 7 – Unwrap

Once the set time has passed, normally at least an hour, you can start to unwrap your body. This is usually done in the reverse order. Unclasp the wraps and allow them to unravel. When you are unwrapped, take a cool shower to rinse off the solution and impurities and then dry off.

How Detox Wraps Work

The detox solution that you are using will be full of clay, minerals r specific herbs that are desired to draw toxins out of your body. While you can use these solutions on their own, using a wrap adds pressure, which increases the chances of absorption. The detox wrap is an active way of getting the toxins to come out of your body, as opposed to the detox bath, which is a passive way.

Chapter 8:

5 Homemade Detox Hair Masks and Shampoos

The hair care industry is raking in billions of dollars every single year but you don't need to contribute to that if you really don't want to. You can easily make your own detox shampoo and hair masks to help remove the toxins and the chemical buildup from your scalp. The following recipes are easy to make and the results will be tremendous.

Shampoos

Use these to cleanse your scalp and effectively get rid of the chemical build up and impurities that are left behind by traditional shampoos and hair care products.

Lemon and Cucumber

The lemon will clean your scalp a treat and the cucumber works to cool and calm things down a little. This is a dead easy recipe to make and is ideal for those who have a dry and itchy scalp.

Ingredients

- 1 fresh lemon, peeled
- 1 fresh cucumber, peeled
- Olive oil – optional
- Rosemary essential oil – optional

Instructions

- Blend the lemon and cucumber in your blender

- Massage into your hair and leave for a few minutes, then rinse out thoroughly

You can add olive oil or rosemary oil blended with the lemon first and then sieved through before blending with the cucumber. If you hair is dry, use more cucumber and if your hair is oily, use more lemon.

Natural pH Balanced Shampoo

If you think the pH levels of your hair are wrong, this shampoo is a great way to put everything back in balance. The recipe is simple to follow and you get all the natural goodness from the ingredients straight to your scalp and hair. The beauty of this recipe is that you can make a large batch and preserve it until you need it.

Ingredients

- 1 can of coconut milk. If you prefer making your own, use about 1 ½ cups

- 1 ¾ cups aloe Vera gel

- Essential oils – optional

Instructions

- Mix the ingredients together with a wire whisk until fully combined

- Pour the mixture out into ice cube trays

- Freeze for a few hours until completely frozen.

- Take one cube out and defrost it thoroughly in a bowl

- Wet your hair and then massage the shampoo into your scalp and gradually work it towards the ends of your hair

- Leave it for 30 seconds or so and then rinse

Do not keep adding more because you cannot see any lather – this recipe does not lather and a little works wonders. You can rinse your hair off using apple cider vinegar as well because this will ensure that all traces are removed. If your ice cubes are large, only use a quarter or half and sore the rest in the refrigerator for up to one week

Coconut Milk Shampoo

Using coconut in your shampoo gives your hair a real treat – plenty of nutrients and fats that will help it to grow. This recipe can also be used as a body wash in the shower.

Ingredients

- 1/3 cup of coconut milk – homemade is best
- ½ cup coconut oil soap
- 2 tsp sweet almond oil
- 10 drops lavender essential oil - optional

Instructions

- Place all the ingredients in a jar and shake well to combine
- Pour out into a squeeze bottle and use as needed
- Shake well before use

Hair Masks

These masks will penetrate deeply into your hair, providing nutrition and an immediate change in the texture and health of your hair.

Aloe and Clay Detox Mask

This recipe calls for bentonite clay and aloe Vera gel to help moisturize your hair. The recipe is easy to follow and inexpensive.

Ingredients

- ½ cup bentonite clay powder
- ½ cup aloe Vera gel

- ¼ cup apple cider vinegar

- 1 extra cup of apple cider vinegar

Instructions

- Mix the clay powder, allow Vera gel and the ¼ cup of apple cider vinegar together until thoroughly combined

- Work it into your hair, massaging it in

- Put a shower cap on and leave it for about 20-30 minutes – do NOT allow it to dry onto your hair

- Rinse it off with 1 cup of apple cider vinegar and leave it for between 1 and 3 minutes before shampooing.

Natural Clay Mud Mask

This is a very simple but highly effective mud mask that can be made with Redmond or bentonite clay> the latter is usually used for detoxing because it has a very powerful drawing effect, pulling toxins out and leaving the hair feeling fresh and new. Essential oils are recommended but be aware that some herbs can darken or lighten your hair. Nettle leaf can be used on any color or type of hair; chamomile flowers are best for light colored hair while rosemary oil is good for dark hair.

For dark hair, mix ¼ cup of rosemary leaf with 2 tbsp. nettle leaf and 2 cups of boiling water. For blonde hair, use 2 tbsp. of nettle leaf and ¼ cup of chamomile flowers in 2 cups of boiling water. Cool and strain into 2 cups

Ingredients

- Herbal tea as per above suggestions

- ½ cup apple cider vinegar

- ¾ cup of Redmond or bentonite clay

- 10 drops of your favorite essential oil – tip – rosemary and lavender oils promote hair growth

Instructions

- Brew the tea and leave it to cool

- Strain thoroughly into t 2 cups

- Pour one cup into the blender and add the apple cider vinegar. If the blades are metal, pour the mixture

into a plastic bowl instead

- Add the clay a bit at a time, mixing well with a non-metal spoon or whisk to incorporate it thoroughly

– the eventual consistency should be like yoghurt

- Add the essential oils and mix them in thoroughly

- Wet your hair and massage a handful of the mixture in,

stating from the roots and going all the way to end of the hair – use as much mixture as needed

- Leave it for between 5 and 20 minutes but do not let it dry

- Rinse with 1 cup of herbal tea mixed with a tbsp. of apple cider vinegar

Chapter 9:
Essential Oils for Body and Mind Detox

Essential oils have been proven time and again to have properties that serve our health, our physical wellbeing and our emotional wellbeing. However, some of them can also act as very powerful detoxification aids for both the body and the mind. These oils can be used alone or mixed as a combination. They must be diluted and can be applied topically on the skin, added to your bah or inhaled. You can also use a diffuse in some cases.

When you use essential oils in your bath water, you must wait until the bath is as full as you want it before you sprinkle in the old – anywhere from 8 to 30 drops, depending on how strong you want it to be. This is because the oils evaporate very quickly and you won't get the full benefit if you add them while the water is running. Do not immerse yourself under the water, as essential oils are irritating to the eyes. Also, if you are using them in the bath, do not use any other soap as some can neutralize the oils and interfere with the way they work.

Some of the best oils, known to have detoxification properties are

- Rose
- Black pepper
- Cypress
- Juniper berry
- Fennel

- Coriander

- Sage

- Parsley

- Frankincense

- Carrot seed

- Grapefruit

- Bitter orange

- Lemon

- Nutmeg

- Peppermint

- Laurel

- Rosemary

- Mandarin

- Hyssop

- Patchouli

- Helichrysum

Always blend your chosen oils in a carrier oil like olive oil, vegetable oil or almond oil before you used them in the bath or on your skin

10 Essential Oils That Will Detox and Purify Your Body

The true beauty of these oils comes in the fact that they have so many different uses, depending on what you need them for. Detoxing is the act of helping to rid the body of all the toxic waste, the negative thoughts you may be having, anxiety, stress and any harmful organisms in the body and these oils contain many benefits.

1. Peppermint Oil

Peppermint oil can be used in a number of ways. First, you can add a few drops to your bath water. Second, you can use it topically; you can add water to a few drops of it and drink it or you can pop a few drops in your detox smoothie or tea.

Peppermint oil is good for helping you to get your concentration levels back up and to maintain them, as well as being soothing for the digestive system. It comes from the peppermint plant, which has been used for medicinal use for thousands of years. It is often mixed with other oils for a true detoxifying blend.

2. Juniper Oil

Juniper oil is derived from the juniper berry, which are also great for the body because of all the antioxidants they contain. They are a great aid for your digestive system and as a diuretic. Using the oil means that you are getting the full essence of the plant without having to use the actual plant.

Juniper oil is good for detoxifying and soothing the mind, to help you alleviate stress and pain. Used as a diuretic, it can flush out toxins and help to get rid of a buildup in water weight, which includes excess sodium.

3. Grapefruit Oil

You may be used to eating grapefruit or drinking grapefruit juice but you may not have known that the oil extracted from the fruit can be of huge help to the body in many ways. One of its properties is that it can help to detoxify the body and it could be the most useful of all the essential oils. Not only that, it does not have to be used just as part of a detox program; grapefruit oil can be used daily to keep your body healthy.

Grapefruit oil has also been scientifically shown to kill off viruses that may be roaming your body, as well as any troublesome microbes. Lastly, it is used as a diuretic, helping to flush toxins and waste out of your body.

4. Rosemary Oil

Maybe you use rosemary as an herb in the kitchen and maybe you just grow it because of its wonderful smell. The oil that comes from the rosemary plant is highly detoxifying, as well as being good for the whole body. If you take the healthy properties of the rosemary plant and put them in an oil, you get the benefits, such an improvement to your digestive system, better circulation, diuretic properties and anti-inflammatory properties.

Rosemary has been shown to fight off memory loss and cancer. It can be inhaled in aromatherapy or you can use it in your bath. You can even add it to massage oil and use it during a massage.

5. Laurel Oil

Laurel oil is derived from the laurel leaf and these have been shown to contain vast amounts of healthy antioxidants that can give your body a boost in more ways than one. Instead of attempting to consume the actual leaf, you get the same benefits from the oil. We all know that one of the top reasons for doing a detox is to get the digestive system moving again and laurel oil does just that; you only need a small amount of it as well. You can also add it to a diffuser to get into your body through the respiratory system.

6. Mandarin Oil

Mandarin oil comes from the fruit and has been shown to have amazing properties in helping to relax and soothe the nervous system. This is one of the best things you can do to get your body back on track and get it prepared to be detoxified. Mandarin oil also helps to purify the blood and can make improvements to your circulatory system.

Because it is derived from the fruit, it has a wonderful aroma and is a nice oil to use in aromatherapy. It helps to boost the function of the liver, which is the single most important organ in your body when it comes to detoxification. If your liver is not performing properly, neither will any of your other organs.

7. Lemon Oil

It has long been known that the lemon has highly astringent properties and is ideal to be used as part of a detoxification plan. Lemon oil is often added to the products you buy for cleaning because it smells nice and promotes a feeling of cleanliness. Some of the benefits of using lemon oil include cancer prevention properties, freeing up the respiratory system and helping the lymphatic system to function correctly. It can also be used as an anti-inflammatory. Lemon oil can be used in a bath, or added to a detox smoothie.

8. Patchouli Oil

Patchouli oil is derived from the plant of the same name and it has been shown to improve, not just your mind but your sex drive as well. Patchouli oil is an essential oil that doesn't get much press but it has some great benefits. It can be used in a detox plan for the body and the mind by adding a few drops to a warm bath. If you want to take advantage of the diuretic properties of patchouli oi, add a few drops to a glass of water, your detox smoothie, soup or tea.

9. Hyssop Oil

Hyssop oil is another one that isn't quite so well-known but, as its benefits become more widely known, it will get more popular. Hyssop oil is used as way of treating problems with the digestive system and that is where you need to start when you detox your body. The digestive system is the part of your body that is responsible for eliminating the most amount of toxins and if it stops working properly, it leaves your body at risk of other conditions and diseases.

10. Helichrysum Oil

You would be forgiven for wondering just how you were going to get more of this highly beneficial plant into your body on a daily basis and that is where helichrysum oil comes into play. Helichrysum is part of the sunflower family and it is chock full of benefits. Many of these target the skin and, as this is the largest organ of the body, it is one of the best for removing toxins. Helichrysum oil is useful for reducing the amount of inflammation in your body and in helping to regenerate cells.

Detox Blends

Not all oils will work the way you want them to and it isn't always easy to find the right blends. This section is designed to give you a few ideas of which oils to blend to help in your detox plan.

One of the most powerful blends of essential oils that is thought to have highly detoxifying effects on all of the organs in your boy, and your skin, is a mix of seaweed oil, juniper berry oil, fennel oil and lemon oil.

Another highly potent mix is fir oil, hyssop oil, fennel oil, patchouli oil and helichrysum oil, blended together with a base oil that is neutral. Live toxicity is often evidenced by pain in the lower and middle back and you may also get bad headaches. This blend of oils is cleansing and should be applied topically to the areas that are toxic. If you are not entirely sure which areas they are, apply it to areas of weakness or use it as an oil for massaging your feet.

A good blend for the lymphatic system and the liver is rosemary oil, geranium oil, roman chamomile oil, carrot seed oil, German chamomile oil, blue tansy oil and helichrysum oil. This potent blend works to cleanse the lymphatic system and the liver removing higher levels of toxins. It can also break up any angry areas in the liver. It should be applied topically, directly over the liver, the solar plexus or used as a full body massage oil.

For stress relief and a mind detox, use a blend of geranium oil, lavender oil, ylang ylang oil, sandalwood oil and blue tansy oil. This special blend helps to free your body of emotional trauma and is also a great blend for a liver detox and in times of distress. Apply topically over the solar plexus, liver and the forehead or use in a foot massage.

Please seek medical advice before you use any of these blends, especially if you are pregnant or are planning to fall pregnant.

Two Feel-Good Essential Oil Recipes

Anti-aging - blend 15 drops of ylang ylang oil with 5 drops of geranium oil into 50 ml of a vegetable oil. Massage it into the neck and face before going to sleep. You can also massage this into your scalp once a week, about 15 minutes before you shampoo your hair.

Anti-stress - this is a blend for a bath. Use 100 ml of a neutral base oil and add 50 drops of lavender oil, 50 drops of mandarin oil and 50 drops if ylang ylang oil. Add to the bath. If you want a tonifying oil, add in 60 drops of lemon oil and 50 drops of rosemary oil.

Bonus Chapters

How to Detox from Alcohol

People who only have the occasional drink will not need to worry about this but for the heavier drinker and those who are diagnosed alcoholics, I hope that this chapter will help you to understand and learn how you can help yourself by undergoing a home detox. Many people don't understand the seriousness of an alcohol detox, or understand how difficult it can be or the dangers of withdrawal.

There are two stages to an alcohol detox; the first starts 6-24 hours after the last drink and can last for up to 7 days. This is the most dangerous period of withdrawal and the person may need medical help. At the very least, they should be properly monitored, especially if this is being done at home, rather than in a detox center. The second stage is the longest and it takes place over a course of months as the brain starts to resume its normal function. It is in this stage when the sleep patterns start to return to normal and emotions come under control.

Preparation for Alcohol Detox at Home

Your Environment

One of the main reasons for wanting to do this in your own home, rather than at a detox center, is for the comfort factor. That's OK but there are certain rules that you must follow. First, you must understand that an alcohol detox and withdrawal does not take all that long but you won't be going anywhere while it's happening. You will have to stay home so make sure you have plenty of books and movies, games to play, whatever it takes to keep your mind off the alcohol. The next rule is, rid your house of all alcohol. There won't be any saving a bit for a special occasion, or keeping it just in case, it all has to go. Once those withdrawal symptoms kick in, you will be heading straight for your emergency stash.

Have a family member of a friend come and stay with you – you are going to need the support from the very first day. They need to be there for at least a few days but manly while you are going through the withdrawal symptoms.

Home remedies for alcohol detox

Dietary Changes

During alcohol detox, there will be times where you won't want to eat or won't be able to keep your food down. However, at this point in time, your diet is absolutely critical. You need to have the right foods and drinks on hand to help you. The idea behind this is the same as someone who is doing a detox diet except it is much more important. You need a house full of fresh fruits and vegetables, whether you like them or not.

This isn't about eating what you like because, if you fill up on moon pies or Cheetos, you are just swapping one problem for another. Instead, the fruits and vegetables are to help speed up the release of the toxins that are rushing around your body. Berries are a good choice have they are full of natural sugars and sugar is something that ex- drinkers want. Oats help to control your blood sugar and help to relax you. Bananas are good sources of energy as well as helping to boost your mood and are full of fiber and potassium. You want foods that are protein rich, like fish, chicken or peanut butter. You don't have to eat huge meals; eat little and often instead.

Don't eat junk or processed food; if you want the best results out of your detox, eat plenty of nutrient rich food. Junk food is full of refined sugar and bad carbohydrate, all increasing the toxins in the body. The idea of the detox is to get rid of these, not add more to them. You may not think that an apple will help you feel better but, trust me, it will in the long run.

Drink enough water

Water is vital to every person, not just those on a detox. You must drink large quantities of water every day but no more than 2 quarts an hour. You can throw a few fresh fruit juices in for a change but, primarily, your fluid intake has to come from water. Your withdrawal symptoms will ease and the toxins will be flushed out of your body that much quicker. Avoid drinking tea or coffee or any other drink that contains caffeine. Your sleep is already going to be disturbed and caffeine will just make that worse. In terms of water, you should be looking at around 100 ounces a day. This will wash the toxins and the chemicals right out of your body, as well as the alcohol and it will also help with the dehydration issues that surround alcohol consumption.

Have enough vitamin B

When you drink alcohol on a daily basis, your levels of vitamin B diminish, causing a deficiency. To help heal your body from the inside, you must make sure you replace that vitamin B as well as taking in sufficient to keep your levels up. You also need to restore vitamin C and magnesium to ensure that your body functions as smoothly as possible.

Use Milk Thistle & Kudzu

Milk thistle extract is a natural way of removing toxins from your body by stopping the liver from absorbing the alcohol and helping to reduce how severe the side effects are. Kudzu has been in use almost since time began as a form of treatment for alcohol consumption. It has powerful antioxidant properties that help to reduce the damage done to the liver and to help it regenerates. 10 grams of kudu powder daily is sufficient to curb the cravings for alcohol.

Use Angelica Extract

Angelica helps to reduce alcohol cravings and the withdrawal symptoms. It's an herb with anti-inflammatory properties that have the power to curb your desire to drink. 5 drops per day is the recommended dosage, added water. It will also help to reduce bloating and headaches that are commonly associated with alcohol abstinence.

Add Cayenne Pepper to Food

Cayenne pepper is another one that helps to curb the cravings and it will increase your appetite as well. Add it food to reduce symptoms of nausea and decreased appetite that come with a withdrawal from alcohol.

Drink Passion Flower Tea

Passion flower tea helps to alleviate interrupted sleep and symptoms of delirium, by relaxing your body and mind. Drink it as often as you want.

Basil

Basil is an extremely potent herb and one of the most effective at reducing cravings. It has both antioxidant and anti- inflammatory properties that help to eliminate free radicals and fully detoxify your body. The best way to take it is to soak fresh basil twigs in water overnight with 20 peppercorns.

Bitter Gourd Leaves

Bitter gourd leaves have been shown to help repair damaged livers. They are packed full of compounds that can help to cure alcoholism through flushing toxins out of the body. The leaves must be ground up to extract the juice and drink fresh in a glass of buttermilk.

Ashwagandha

Ashwagandha is one of those ancient herbs that are full of medicinal properties. It has both anti-oxidant and anti- inflammatory properties that help to detox the body while improving brain function at the same time. It can help to alleviate tension, stress and help you to feel better overall. Take one teaspoon with a glass of milk two time a day.

Gotu Kola

This is a supplement that helps to improve the functions of the brain and the nervous system. It also acts as a blood purifier, keep stress at bay and reduce anxiety. 50 grams should be taken three times a day.

All of these home remedies help to keep your stamina up so that you can better fight off the addiction and beat the withdrawal symptoms. As you can see from the list, most of these are included the detox diets we talked about earlier and can all help to rush the toxins out of the body much quicker than they would come out otherwise. The quicker the toxins leave, the quicker you will begin to feel better. Make no mistake though; the path to alcohol recovery is much longer than detoxing your body for a week but with the right help and support, this is one battle that you can win.

Dealing with Cravings

It is normal to experience cravings, they are part and parcel of any addiction and you will be keenly aware of them throughout withdrawal. They can also appear many weeks or months, even years in some cases, after you have kicked the habit. The following are some important facts about cravings that you need to know to learn how to deal with them:

What You Should Know About Cravings:

Cravings are not caused through a lack of motivation or willpower. They also do not mean that your withdrawal and detox is not working. Cravings actually last for a very short period of time and they are never there 24/7. What triggers cravings is some kind of emotional or physical upset or discomfort and managing that will help you to manage your cravings.

Things You Can Do to Manage Cravings:

You need to know what triggers a craving. It could be a person, a place, or something that reminds you of alcohol. Once you learn to identify the triggers, you need to learn to direct your mental energy elsewhere, to ways that will help you to avoid those triggers again.

Tell yourself constantly why you have stopped drinking and list down the negative effects of the alcohol on your life. List the positives to giving it up and staying clean as well.

Call on your support network for help when you need it.

Make sure you follow the home remedies for an alcohol detox. Detoxing your body will help these cravings to disappear quicker.

After the Alcohol Detox

About 36 hours into your detox, you will begin to feel very uncomfortable and irritable; this will last for up to a week. Do not, under any circumstances, stop your detox. In fact, at this stage, it is more important than ever that your diet is right and that you are maintaining your health and your detox routine. Make sure you are taking any vitamins and supplements that you need, getting a little exercise and sleeping.

It won't take long before you are able to get back to normal as long as you are not placed under any stress. What you have to understand here is that you have detoxed from the alcohol. The toxins are gone but, if you don't make significant changes to your lifestyle, you will soon be back where you started.

Once the alcohol is gone from your system, you will find that your appetite increases. This is where you should follow the detox guidelines up above to ensure that your body stays healthy and fit enough for you to fight off any cravings. You will also probably be very malnourished and will need to eat good whole foods to get your strength back up. Again, as I said before, eat small and often rather than trying to struggle though a big meal. Just make sure you are eating the right foods.

If this is the very first time you have had to go through an alcohol detox, be glad it is over. Learn from it and never put yourself back in the situation where you have to do it again. The principles of an alcohol detox are no different from any other detox; it is just a much harder experience to go through.

Don't Forget Your Pets

When we talk about detoxing, we always talk in terms of humans and we tend to forget about our pets. We all have a pretty good idea what toxins are and we also have an understanding of how they affect our health. We know that they can worsen any existing health problems but do you know how much the toxins that affect you affect your pets? The problem with toxins is that they are hidden and we are unwittingly causing both our animals and ourselves health problems that are not necessary. We already know how bad toxins are for us but, for your pets, they can be devastating, for a number of reasons.

First, your pets are smaller than you are and they have much smaller livers, kidneys and lungs, all the organs that help to eliminate the toxins. When they are exposed to toxins, those organs have to work so much harder to remove them. Second, they don't live as long as we do. They don't have the time for their bodies to eliminate those toxins on a gradual basis. They can't talk to us, tell us that something they are eating or breathing in is making them ill. They can't change their own food or stop using a cleaning fluid or spray that is irritating their lungs. They rely on us, their owners, 100% because we control the environment they live in and the food they eat.

So, how do you minimize the toxins that your pet is exposed to and help them to get rid of the ones they already have in their bodies? Before we look at how you can help them, let's take a deeper look at these toxins and how our cats and dogs come into contact with them.

Tracking the Toxins

There are several ways that your pet can be exposed to toxins. Some are through accidental ingestion. Weed killers, exhaust fumes, pesticides, motor oil, and chemical deicers get into our pets when they walk on grass, paths or roads, when they at grass coated in chemicals and lick dust and dirt off their coats and their paws. The air fresheners, household cleaners, washing products and any other chemical that we use in the household can also find their way into your pet's body. Toxins in the water, in commercially prepared dog foods and treats and in medications and shampoos we use on them. Some toxins are actually produced in their bodies, like ammonia, through their own metabolic processes or through bacteria or yeast in the GI tract.

In the wild, animals have a more efficient elimination system for flushing out toxins. These systems have developed over the years to counteract natural toxins in the environments they frequent but domesticated pets don't have the ability to combat the constant bombardment of toxins that they are faced with on a daily basis, mainly because their bodies have not had the years they need in which to adapt enough to fight the battle.

What Are The Ill Effects of Toxins?

When a body is healthy, the toxins are quickly eliminated through the lungs, kidneys and liver, as well as the intestines and the skin. Because domesticated pets have not adapted their elimination systems to cope with the sheer numbers of toxins, they react in pretty much the same way as we do – their bodies become inflamed, and they up their production of mucus or diarrhea to try to help the immune system to get rid of them.

When a body takes in too many toxins, it has to store the excess until there is a good time to get rid of them. For many pets, that good time will never come and the toxins simply continue to build up. Over time, you might notice that your dog or cat is lethargic, fatigues and prone to infections. The overload of toxins will eventually stop the immune system from working to the extent where they begin to suffer with tumors and cysts and, as the cells degrade even further, even more serious health problems will begin to manifest themselves.

There is good news though, most animals are perfectly well equipped to fight infection and disease, eliminate some toxins and to restore their internal organs and systems back to health but they do need your help. If you feed your pet a natural diet, with plenty of exercise and rest and playtime thrown in for good measure your pet will have a level of health that you would never have thought possible. In short, you can give them a new lease of life by following the 15 steps below to detoxing your pet.

Fifteen Steps to Detox Your Pet

Give them better quality food and treats

This is always your first port of call in proving the life and longevity of your pet. If you feed your pet on cheap supermarket brand foods, you are feeding them chemicals, in the form of additives, artificial flavoring and coloring. Commercial foods also contain low quality fillers and proteins that are hard on your pet's digestive system, as well as increasing the toxins in the body. Instead, go for high quality natural foods and treats. It may be more expensive but you cannot put a price on your pet's life.

Only Filtered Water

While your tap water may be classed as fit to drink, it is full of toxins, in the form of certain minerals and metals, along with the chemicals that are added to keep it clean – chlorine and fluoride for starters. There are even going to be trace amounts of compounds that are similar to hormones and a number of other suspicious things that will harm the health of your pet. Water filtration units are not expensive and you can buy them almost anywhere.

Add Herbs and Nutrient Supplements

There are lots of herbs and natural supplements that you can add to your pet's food that will help cleanse their systems. Lots of these nutrients are usually missing from commercially prepared foods, such as amino acids, antioxidants, chlorophyll, essential fatty acids and trace minerals. Do your homework and find good quality supplements with cleansing herbs that will help your dog to live a longer and healthier life.

Cut out Household Chemicals

As well as the obvious ones, such as fly sprays, cleaning chemicals and solvents, there are also toxins fond in perfumes, deodorants, air fresheners, plug in air fresheners, washing products and tumble dryer sheets. These tend to be full of chemicals that are not regulated and are not tested by health protection agencies and many of them have been prove to have an adverse effect on breathing problems in both people and pets. Either use only 100% natural products or make your own. Ingredients like lemon, vinegar, and baking soda all make excellent cleaning products and they are all natural and non-toxic.

Exercise Every Day

You need to get your body moving to help eliminate toxins and so does your pet. Exercise speeds up the elimination process by moving waste products through the digestive tract. It also improves blood and lymph fluid circulation, which are the two main means your pet uses for moving debris and toxins through the body. Exercises also help to improve respiration, which allows the excess toxins to be removed from the respiratory tract. If you can't get out for a walk with them every day, make sure you give them exercise in other ways by playing with them in the garden – and that includes the cat!

Improve the Quality of the Air

Pollution can come from all directions and indoors it comes from household cleaner chemicals, perfumes, deodorants, air fresheners and cigarette or cigar smoke. It can also come from synthetic furnishings like carpets, cushion covers or flooring, even the furniture itself. If your new furniture is giving off the aroma of "new", make sure you keep your pets away from the areal and keep windows open to ventilate the area well. You can also use window fans and bathroom fans to remove the effects of hairspray and perfume, or other things that you regularly spray around.

Minimize the Amount of Outdoor Chemicals they are Exposed to

If your pets spend time outside, they will come into contact with a number of different chemicals – pest control, fertilizers, weed killers and much more. If your dog eats grass, watch them while you are out walking, especially in public places where chemicals are likely to have been used. You can eliminate this behavior by adding in greens to their food, both cats and dogs. You can actually grow cat grass, which is free of the toxic contaminants.

Reduce the Amount of Conventional Medications You Use

There are a lot of toxic chemicals and compounds in traditional treatments for fleas and ticks, not to mention worm tablets and vaccines, as well as lots of other drugs that your pet may need. While these treatments may be a necessary part of owning a pet, you can keep in check how much they are exposed to. Don't over dose them on the flea and tick treatments, only administer medications when it is absolutely necessary and, where you can look for alternative treatments. For example, using lemons, rosemary and water and spraying it once a week can make a good flea and tick treatment. It's also much cheaper than having to use what your veterinary practitioner sells. Think about the vaccines your dog has every year – it doesn't actually need them and it has been proven that they are not necessary and can be dangerous to the health of your pet, as well as decreasing their lifespan naturally.

Support their Liver

The liver is the main vehicle used for eliminating toxins, not just in humans but in animals too. Make sure your pet has the right antioxidants in his or her diet as these help the liver to work more efficiently. Use herbs like milk thistle, added to their food every day, to boost the liver function. While your pet is young and healthy, it probably won't need any liver support but older animals and those that are on medications will do. Please make sure you speak with a holistic vet before giving your dog or cat anything as he or she is trained to advise you what you should, or shouldn't as the case may be, using.

Provide Support for the Immune System

In the same way that yours does, your pet's immune system works with their organs to keep them well. To support their immune system, you are helping to keep their lungs, liver, kidneys and intestines healthy as well as their skin so that their natural detoxification system will work properly. If you want your pets to be healthy, feed them a high quality mineral and multivitamin supplement, one that is designed for pets, not humans. For older pets or those that are very active, you can also give them pet antioxidant supplements.

Help their Skin to Breathe

Cats and dogs use their skin to eliminate toxins and regular brushing helps it to breathe, which allows the toxins to come out. It also gets rid of any dust and rubbish that may accumulated on their coats, debris that could contain chemical residues, thus making sure your reduce the amount of toxins ingested when they groom themselves. For dogs, look at the bathing products you are using. Are they high quality, made from natural products? Always use natural grooming products to cut down on the amount of toxins your pet take in when you are bathing him or her.

Don't forget, although they remove toxins through their skin, it is also a way in.

Support Their Digestive System

When your pet digests toxins, many of them are eliminated through the colon and keeping their digestive system healthy means that the toxins move n before they get the chance to do any damage to the walls of the intestines or are reabsorbed back into the body. If your pet has a sluggish or irritated bowel, he or she may have chronic diarrhea and this suggests that something is not right inside. If your pet is constipated, the toxins can go back into their blood before they can be eliminated, further complicating the problem. Bacteria and yeast are capable of producing toxins, which can have an adverse effect so make sure you give your pet probiotics, enzymes or a complete supplement that is designed to support the gastrointestinal system.

Support Their Kidneys

The easiest and simplest thing to do to help support your pet's kidneys in make sure they are drinking sufficient amounts of filtered water daily. Toxins that are eliminated through the kidneys can be highly concentrated if your pet is dehydrated and this can damage the structures that make up the filtration system in the kidneys. Also, mineral particles form if the urine is concentrated, which could result in crystals or stones form that can block up or irritate the urinary tract. This can be the start of numerous infections that simply won't go away or keep coming back. If your dog or cat is not a big drinker, add water or broth into their food. Cats in particular will drink very little so keep them on a high quality wet diet where possible. If you feed them on the pouches or cans of food, add a little warm water to the pouch or can afterwards and add it to the food. Not only does this increase their hydration, it also ensures that they are getting all of the goodness out of the food because none of the jelly or gravy is left behind.

Keep Things Clean

The home environment has been shown to have far worse air quality than outdoors. However, a certain mount of the toxins in our houses comes in from outdoors as dust or other pollutants. Dust, vacuum and clean regularly to keep these toxins down and reduce the amount of toxic matter that your pet can ingest. Also, be very strict about cleaning their beds on a regular basis and their food and water bowls.

Use Herbs and Homeopathic Remedies to Help Your Pet Detox

Because they live with us and because we are responsible for their wellbeing, it is up to us to keep the levels of the toxins down. However, all pets can benefit from regular and gentle detoxing, which you can do with the aid of herbs and other homeopathic remedies that can help to support their organs, cleanse their systems and help them to eliminate toxins better. Again, please seek advice from a registered holistic vet before you give your pet any supplements.

Rules of the Detox Diet

As you probably know by now, there are several different meanings to the word "detox", all of which differ based on the affect they have on your body. One of the most popular goals of a detox program is to purify the body and cleanse it of all of the unclean toxins that it has become infested by during our normal routines.

This buildup of toxicity in your body is obviously something to be alarmed about. After all, any foreign toxic chemical simply being present in your body in trace amounts is enough to send anybody to the doctor, or at least make a major shift in their lifestyle choices in order to facilitate a healthier body. However, although serious, the buildup of toxic chemicals that detoxification is supposed to reverse should not come as a surprise to you given the way we live our lives in today's modern day and age, an age where once widely accepted traditions of health are now ignored for the sake of convenience.

In our normal every day routines what do we eat? Processed sugars, preservatives, corn syrup, saturated fats, such chemicals that we would be averse to should we see them in their true form are eaten in large quantities because they make the food we eat and the beverages we drink taste better. Eating fast food has become a regular, every day portion of our lives, we actually eat these poisonous foods for fun! Even when we eat at home, we often accompany our drinks with carbonated beverages or alcohol.

When not consuming alcohol with meals, we often consume it for enjoyment whilst socializing. Getting heavily inebriated due to the consumption of alcohol has become an extremely common past time for the average person in today's modern day and age.

Additionally, we fuel our increasingly work oriented and fast paced lives through the use of stimulants such as caffeine and nicotine, the latter of which often brings with it substances as toxic as tar and cyanide due to the method via which it is most commonly consumed. Caffeine providing beverages and foods are not all that much better, for they obstruct your body's natural system as well.

With all of these unimaginably toxic substances being pumped by us into our very own bodies, willingly at that, it should not come as a surprise that these toxins build up in our bodies and prevent it from functioning the way it should.

The best way to fix this problem is via a detox diet which not only cuts you off from all of these poisonous chemicals, it also makes you eat the kinds of foods that allow your body to cleanse itself and clean out all of the toxins from within it more efficiently.

Here is a list of some of the rules you will need to be following while you are on your detox diet:

> Complete avoidance of all stimulants and depressants: This one should be pretty obvious but equally difficult to follow. After all,

tobacco and alcohol are such intrinsic parts of our lives, even after the almost worldwide vilification of tobacco products after it was discovered that they caused cancer. It's not your fault if you can't decrease your intake of these products, but you need to realize that they are responsible for a lot of the damage that your body is suffering, as they introduce some of the most toxic chemicals into your body out of perhaps any other substances that we consume. If you are addicted to either cigarettes or alcohol, or if you feel as though they have become an unavoidable part of your social life, it's best not to quit cold turkey because you will just end up relapsing within a day or two, perhaps three if you have sufficient will power. The better option to pursue in this scenario is to gradually decrease the quantity that you consume. For example, if you generally drink four glasses of beer a day try decreasing the amount by one glass per week or even half a glass. The same technique can be used for cigarettes as well. Interestingly, although caffeine is a stimulant, it's actually an important part of your detox diet as you will see in list entry number 9.

Complete avoidance of all processed and chemically altered foods: Another no brainer, but this one should be relatively easy to accomplish at least when compared to the one before it. However, don't think that just because the media doesn't tell you they're bad doesn't mean that you don't get addicted to foods that have been processed or chemically altered. These foods positively affect your mood similar to the way very mild drugs do, and your body can get used to that. However, working these foods out of your daily life is fairly simple. The first thing you need to do, of course, is to cut out all fast food and just eating out in general. Cook food at home, make sure that the ingredients you use aren't processed and don't contain any chemical additives and you'll be good to go. You'll even really like this new diet of yours because it will begin to taste so good once you start to enjoy the real flavors of food rather than chemicals that provide you with a false sense of taste! Soda might be more difficult to quit since it is very addictive but using the same tactic you used with alcohol or cigarettes will definitely get the job done.

An increase in the intake of vegetables and fruits: Out goes the bad, in goes the good, this is the basic rule of any detox diet worth its salt and any detox diet that does not encourage this mindset will never be anything more than a hoax! The good that must go in is mostly fruits and vegetables based. Out of all of the foods that you can possibly eat, none are better for you than vegetables or fruits because they have absolutely everything that you could possibly want from your food! From vitamins to minerals to fiber, even protein if you eat the right vegetables, fruits and vegetables should ideally be all that your detox diet consists of but even just making these foods a regular part of your regular meals will make a huge difference. This is because, apart from the aforementioned vitamins, minerals etc. that fruits and vegetables contain, they also contain antioxidants. Antioxidants are chemicals that detoxify your body and get rid it of pretty much all of the toxic chemicals that are making it such an inefficient and unhealthy place. This means that the more fruits and vegetables you eat, the faster you will detoxify! Just don't overdo it because too much of anything can never be good.

A decrease in the intake of meat: Meat is an important part of the modern diet. The vast majority of people that are living in today's modern day and age incorporate a large amount of meat into their diets, to the point where the average modern meal is based around a meat related entree, with vegetables serving as side dishes and fruits little more than oft forgotten after thoughts. We can't really be blamed for this, after all meat tastes so good! However, red meat especially can clog up your system because it has a lot of saturated fat which is a chemical that can become quite toxic if you consume too much of it. Kicking the meat habit will be incredibly difficult, but as long as you cut down on red meat, reducing it to one serving a day, you will be able to detox your body successfully, as long as your fruit and vegetable intake is comparably high. If you quit meat, you can use nuts in order to supplement your protein intake. You can derive your entire daily requirement of protein entirely from nuts and legumes, which will allow you to stay healthy, possibly bulk up, and avoid saturated fats altogether!

Start buying organic: The way we grow foods has become increasingly warped. There was once a time when farming was just that: farming. Some crops were lost, some grew bad, but most grew normally and these crops were both delicious and healthy. Nowadays, however, farming is done on an industrial scale, which means that the same old methods that farmers once used simply won't cut it anymore. Farming now involves the spraying of pesticides and insecticides in order to make sure that every single crop makes it and is harvested, and you can imagine how dangerous these chemicals are when consumed. Hence, while detoxing it is extremely important to buy organic fruits and vegetables, and even meat, because these foods will not have any chemicals used to treat them at any stage of the manufacturing process. The vegetables and fruits will not have been grown in chemically treated fertilizer, they would not have been sprayed with poison to prevent them from being lost to plague, and this means that you will not be filling your body with poisons while you are on this diet, giving your body time to heal itself.

Eat raw as much as possible: This rule is part of the "good comes in" half of the detox motto. There are some foods that absolutely cannot be eaten raw, foods like potatoes, eggs and, of course, meat. However, there are a lot more foods that absolutely can be eaten raw, including the vast majority of vegetables as well as practically every fruit in existence, and it is important to eat these foods raw as much as you can. This is because of a little known fact: cooking drains foods of its nutrients. It kills germs and other microbes, but the heat from cooking also kills organic matter such as vitamins that reduces the nutritional effectiveness of the food that you are eating. Cooking also kills antioxidants, which as you will remember from a few rules ago are instrumental in helping you detoxify your system as fast as possible. Hence, in order to get the maximum nutritional benefit from the detox foods that you are eating, eat them raw! Also, try to avoid food that needs to be cooked. It's not that it's bad for you, it's just that there is not better diet than a raw vegan diet, so try to follow this diet if you want extremely effective results!

Drink as much water as possible: Water is the key to life. We can survive for days without food, indeed after a while we can even forget our hunger because our survival response kicks in and starts using up fat to keep us alive. However, we cannot survive more than a day or two without water, and the time we spend without water will be nothing more than pure agony. There is an important reason why this is so, and that is that water powers our body in every single way possible. Every liquid substance in our body needs water to exist, water exists somewhere in the process of the creation of that substance, from blood to bile to spit. Without water, these substances cannot replenish themselves. This means that your body will weaken and will be unable to fully utilize the detoxifying foods that you are eating. Additionally, water really cleans up your system in a meaningful and efficient way. Just like how it helps clean virtually everything, water

speeds up your metabolism and allows your body to use it to dilute the toxic substances within it to tolerable levels that makes them much easier to expel via excretion. The best way to increase your water intake is to replace your beverages with water. Instead of juice or soda, have water and get healthier for it!

Go for better grain choices: The types of grain that we eat are incredibly important because grains are not immune to the immense refinement that undergoes practically every type of food that we eat. The bread that we eat is usually made of refined flour that is what allows it to possess its white color and firm and consistent texture and shape. Real bread is supposed to be lumpy, it's supposed to be rough, in essence it's supposed to be exactly what it is: *real* bread. If you want to avoid toxic chemicals that would make you feel terrible by clogging up your entire system, the best thing that you can do is to avoid refined grains. Whether it's pasta or bread or any other food that is derived from a grain, make sure it's made from whole grain. Try to get bread that is as unprocessed as possible. Really, the only process that should go into the making of your bread is the baking itself, without which the bread wouldn't really be bread at all!

Drink coffee and tea in moderation: This may come across as somewhat odd considering the fact that stimulants are supposed to be bad for you. However, it is not the stimulants themselves but the chemicals they often bring with them that cause the harm. Nicotine, for example, is not that bad, but the cigarettes that are used to consume it contain tar and cyanide, two chemicals that you really don't want inside your body. Caffeine is actually not bad for you at all, the only real damage that it can do is upset your circadian rhythm and interrupt your sleep patterns, along with potentially getting you addicted to the point where you can't really get up without it. However, coffee and tea also possess antioxidants, and plenty of them. Tea especially is an enormous source of antioxidants, so try to consume it when you can. However, don't overdose on either of these beverages because the side effects, such as jitteriness and insomnia, are nothing to sneeze at!

Find alternates to dairy products: Dairy products are such a widely accepted part of our lives that we can barely even imagine a situation where drinking milk was not really good for your health. To be fair, milk is a great source of calcium and vitamin D, and is especially important in children that are in their growing phase. However, cow's milk is often treated using chemicals, and it is nearly impossible to get cow's milk that has not been chemically treated. Indeed, cow's milk that has not been treated is actually not safe to drink. Additionally, cow's milk is not designed for human consumption, and so our digestive system doesn't really agree with it. While you are on your detox diet, go for soymilk instead. It is better for your digestive system, can be found without any chemical treatment and is chock full of antioxidants to help you flush out the toxic chemicals from your body!

Chapter 10:

When is Detoxing Necessary?

I n order to understand in which situations detoxification becomes necessary, one must first understand what exactly detoxification is supposed to accomplish. This helps provide a more balanced understanding of the subject that is very important while moving forward with the detoxification process.

Detoxification, through its removal of toxic substances from your body, improves your health, this much is true, but what it also does is that it helps you overcome some of your most destructive addictions.

This is because when your body becomes used to the toxic substances it now has within it, mostly due to the fact that these chemicals make it feel good, you become addicted to certain substances.

This means that detoxification pertains not just to specific diets intended to purge your body of toxins, it also refers to processes by which you can kick habits and addictions.

Cigarette Addiction

One example of a detoxification process is when you stop smoking. Your body has become so used to the nicotine that it has started to consider tar and cyanide to be feel good chemicals as well, which means that when you quit smoking you are going to feel certain symptoms These symptoms are called withdrawal. It is when your body is so dependent on certain drugs that it considers these substances to be healthy parts of what it needs in order to function properly. This means that when you quit cigarettes, you are going to experience withdrawal.

Certain symptoms of withdrawal include a loss of appetite, insomnia, irritability and just a general distaste for everything because all you want from your life while you are detoxing from cigarettes is, well, a cigarette. Quitting cold turkey is very possible, but bear in mind that it is going to be a somewhat uncomfortable process particularly if you are not especially strong willed.

Cigarette smoking is one of the most prevalent addictions in the world, despite the fact that it is widely known that smoking cigarettes will almost certainly cause cancer, whether in the lungs or in the mouth, in the long run. This goes to show just how incredibly addictive the stuff is, and how difficult it is to quit it.

Smoking becomes a part of our social gatherings, it becomes a part of how we bond with our bosses, becomes a part of how we deal with stress and anxiety in general. A large amount of people in the world, when faced with a problem that causes stress or seems insurmountable, deal with the situation right after they have smoked a cigarette and calmed their nerves.

However, when you quit smoking you will find that your overall health will start to appreciate considerably. Your lung capacity will increase as will your stamina, you will probably be able to become a lot more sexually active, your body will start absorbing nutrients in a much more efficient way and just in general you will start feeling a lot better than you did while you were smoking.

This is because your body recognizes that tar and cyanide are poisonous but ignores their presence due to the fact that they bring nicotine with them. Once you stop giving your body nicotine, it will start to clean house automatically by purging itself of all of these toxic chemicals Hence, quitting cigarettes and allowing your body time to evacuate itself of the toxic chemicals is one example of detoxification. If you are addicted to cigarettes, even if the addiction consists of two or three a day at the moment, you need to detox in order to prevent sinking into deeper addiction.

Alcohol Addiction

There are few substances in the world that are as destructive as alcohol. It is immensely addictive, and the worst part is that it is socially accepted as well which means that it is very easy to fall into the trap of alcohol addiction.

There is a limit to how much alcohol is acceptable. Having a beer or two, a glass of wine or a glass of whiskey while you are out with friends is alright because it does not introduce so much of the stuff that when you stop it would cause withdrawal.

However, when you start drinking every single day you will find that that is the start of a slippery slope that is very difficult to climb back up from. Doing anything every day gives your body the impression that it is a part of your daily diet and it slowly becomes dependent on that chemical.

What alcohol dependency does is that it makes you unable to deal with anxiety or stress without it. Additionally, people that are addicted to alcohol find that they are also unable to go to sleep without having a drink or two.

If you get to this point, you can be sure that you are on that slippery slope to alcohol addiction. However, frequent detoxes can help you ensure that you do not become dependent on alcohol because your body will be used to long periods where you do not consume the substance.

That is all an alcohol detox is really. An extended period of time where you do not consume any form of alcohol, whether at a party or at night in order to sleep. If you feel as though you are unable to cope with your emotions without alcohol, you probably have an addiction.

Keep in mind that a detox from alcohol would only really work if you drink at most four beers, two glasses of wine or a glass of whiskey every day. Any more than that and you are almost certainly addicted and will be unable to detox cold turkey without causing severe discomfort to yourself.

This is mostly due to the fact that your body has probably become utterly independent on the substance. Hence, if you drink a drink or two a day, go for the detox. If it's more than that, get yourself into alcoholics anonymous.

Drug Addiction

Addiction to drugs is one of the most severe epidemics in recent history. Ever since the invention of hardcore, refined drugs such as heroin and crystal meth, the amount of drug addicts has massively increased in recent times, to the point where millions of people are now addicted to hard drugs.

Hard drugs are not the only things that people are getting addicted to. Medicines that are often prescribed to people by their own doctors can be considered incredibly addictive due to the immense amounts of serotonin that they release within your brain in order to have their effect.

Drugs such as oxycodone, hydrocodone, vicodin and especially morphine, the unaltered and legal version of heroin, are incredibly addictive, and it should come as no surprise to you that all of these drugs are pain killers. Painkillers are, after all, placebos that give your brain a positive buzz to focus on instead.

This often happens when people are prescribed with painkillers following a surgery or an injury of some kind that has left them with pain. Doctors often give their patients an unlimited supply of these painkillers in order to help them deal with the pain that they are feeling.

However, this has the effect of making these people dependent on the drug, with the dependence working much in the same way that alcohol dependence does. When people get off the painkillers, they are sometimes unable to deal with pain at all because they are so used to using the painkillers to dull the sensation.

Hence, a lot of people end up addicted to these powerful painkillers and experience symptoms of withdrawal if they are not able to continue using these drugs. In this way an addiction is born, a process of detoxification becomes necessary.

Our body needs to learn how to deal with pain naturally again, which means that we need to rid it of all of these toxins in order to teach it to do that once more. The detox procedure works in exactly the same way, you just stop taking the drug entirely until you no longer need it.

However, in cases where you are addicted to heroin, crystal meth or have a severe dependence on prescription drugs, trying to quit cold turkey would end up causing you severe discomfort. Indeed, trying to completely stop using hard drugs such as heroin after you have developed a dependency for them can even result in your death, so it is important that you proceed with caution. If you feel as though you are dependent to a dangerous degree on these drugs, go and see a therapist and try your best to get yourself into narcotics anonymous.

In situations where the number of times you have tried hard drugs is still in the single digits, or situations where your use of prescription drugs is starting to or has recently started to get out of control, going on a detox and avoiding the substance can be the best way to get past your growing addiction.

Fast Food Addiction

An addiction to fast food is not usually what people have in mind when they picture addictions. However, fast food addictions are even more prevalent than drug addictions, and are extremely dangerous for one's health even if there is no chance of dying because of an overdose caused by fast food.

Fast food addiction is real because it is not normal food. Fast food is mass produced and heavily altered by chemicals in order to make it taste unnaturally good which helps our bodies ignore the fact that it is almost entirely junk which holds little to no nutritional value for our bodies.

These chemicals trigger a response in your brain that is shockingly similar to the one you get from consuming moderate level drugs. Your brain begins releasing dopamine and serotonin, two chemicals called the "feel good" chemicals because they are released whenever your body is doing anything that makes you feel pleasure.

This results in your body associating unhealthy fast food with a reward response within your brain and begins to crave it in increasing amounts. Nowadays, it is not uncommon for the average family to eat out two or three times a week. Certain people even eat fast food every single day, and there is a special group of people which certain fast food giants like to call "super heavy users" who eat more than one meal a day at a fast food place.

An addiction to fast food is incredibly dangerous because of the low nutritional value that fast food holds. Little to no vitamins or minerals, often not nearly enough fiber or carbohydrates and definitely no antioxidants whatsoever make fast food a terrible way to eat. What fast food does have are copious amounts of saturated fat, processed sugar in spades and protein since all fast food is basically meat.

Eating such a toxic cocktail of chemicals can result in obesity and diabetes, not to mention high cholesterol and blood pressure, heart palpitations, sleep apnea and the occasional heart attack. Regularly eating fast food is a recipe for death and nothing else, and harms you just as much in the long run as hard drugs even though the short term effects are not as severe.

Quitting fast food is a lot easier than quitting hard drugs or alcohol, however. The level of addiction has not yet reached the point where foodaholics anonymous has become a thing, and we should all be thankful for that, and so quitting fast food cold turkey will probably not cause you any real pain.

However, you should keep in mind that quitting fast food would cause certain withdrawal symptoms such as depression and sexual dysfunction. This is because your body is used to a mild high that you get after eating fast food and would crave it. However, you will not experience any severe form of discomfort and your health will improve within a few weeks of having quit fast food. Indeed, within days of quitting the stuff you won't even remember why you liked it so much.

Fast food addiction is a serious issue, and detoxing from these poisonous and toxic foods is essential if we want to improve our overall health and make for ourselves a brighter future.

Once your body is no longer addicted to fatty foods and sugary drinks you will feel your energy levels going up and will feel fresher throughout the day, all thanks to the fact that you detoxed from fast food in the first place.

The aforementioned addictions can all be treated to some extent using a process of detoxification. As long as your drug addiction is not too severe, quitting cold turkey is the best way to allow your body to rid itself of the chemicals that it has accumulated over the course of an unhealthy life.

Detoxing also tells you an important thing about yourself: it allows you to ascertain whether you are addicted or not. If you smoke on occasion or fairly regularly, if you drink every day, if you eat at a fast food place very often, even if you partake in hard drugs from time to time, you might be telling yourself that you are not addicted, that you can quit absolutely any time you want.

Detoxing is the way you can put yourself to the test. Try to go without your choice of drug for three days and your body will tell you if you are addicted or not. If you are unable to deal with stress or anxiety or start suffering from insomnia, you can be sure that you are addicted. If you start experiencing withdrawal symptoms, your detox will have told you something extremely important about the things that you are addicted to.

Chapter 11:

When Can Detoxing Be Dangerous?

The people doing the detoxing rather than the process of detoxing itself cause the dangers of detoxing most often. Remember, detoxing is a natural process whereby you purge your body of dangerous substances and toxins in order to help it function in a more efficient manner and improve your overall health.

However, much like any good tool, detoxing must be used in a proper manner. There are detox diets out there that are endorsed by big name celebrities, celebrities who probably don't use these diets themselves and are just doing the endorsements for the money that could cause some major damage to body.

Also, there is such a thing as "too much of a good thing". Detoxing too much can be dangerous as well, particularly if detoxing involves overdosing on a single food that supposedly helps in the detox process and ignoring all of the other equally important areas of your nutrition that you begin to neglect. Doing so will result in nutritional deficiencies which can develop into serious problems if they are not addressed.

In order to help you detox in a safer manner, here are some ways in which detoxing can become dangerous:

> Restriction of nutrients: Certain detox diets encourage you to avoid certain nutrients because they supposedly cause a buildup of toxic chemicals within your system. You need to keep in mind that toxic chemicals are not caused by the consumption of nutrients. Nutrients are just what they are, nutrients, and toxic

chemicals and nutrients are never the same thing. Avoiding certain nutrients can cause severe problems such as malnutrition. You are going on a detox diet to improve your health, and avoiding any kind of nutrient will be detrimental to your health in some way or another.

Restriction of calories: A lot of detox diets encourage you to lower your calorie intake. There is absolutely no reason that you have to do this. Reducing one's intake of calories is important if you want to lose weight, not if you want to detoxify your body. Reducing calorie intake can result in deterioration of your health, especially if it's done to an extreme extent to the point where you are going hours without eating. This is actually the opposite of what you should actually be doing.

Liquid based diets: These diets are another example of what is wrong with the industry that has been built around detox diets. A thing that is meant to improve people's health is now being used to earn money, but such is the way of the world and there is little we can do about it apart from learn to avoid these diets. Liquid diets can be extremely dangerous for your health because liquid foods don't provide the same fiber content and nutritional value as solid foods and liquid diets virtually never provide enough protein. Hence, avoiding liquid diets is the best way for you to keep your health sound while detoxing. Make a special effort to avoid diets that encourage you to consume only water, as these diets will completely wreck your system and severely lower the quality of your health.

Shortcut diets: There is no such thing as a shortcut to good health, and any diet that is using that line to coax you into buying it is definitely not worth your time. Such products are a part of the problem, actually, because they put it into people's minds that the process of detoxing can be accomplished within an extremely short span of time and thus is not worth investing a lot of time into. These diets also involve a lot of shortcuts such as calorie counting that makes you lose weight and thus would make you feel as though you are detoxing. Remember, detoxing has absolutely nothing to do with weight. It is supposed to flush your body of internal toxins and help make you feel good. It will make your skin glow but it is certainly not supposed to make you lose weight, so if a diet offers you a shortcut to getting a clean internal system, avoid that diet like the plague.

Diets that aren't detox diets at all: Detoxing has become the name of a product now that companies have wizened up to the fact that detox diets are incredibly effective and are thus become incredibly popular, especially in recent times. However, these companies don't know the first thing about what a detox diet is supposed to do, they assume that it is just like any other diet and is supposed to make you lose weight. Hence, avoid these diets that big name companies offer you. In essence, this rule is an amalgamation of all of the rules before it. Detoxing is supposed to be relaxing and help you feel good, not make you sick!

Now that you have gotten a general idea of what kinds of detox procedures can be dangerous, you also need to keep in mind the previous chapter. Detoxing from hard drugs can be extremely dangerous, especially if you have become dependent on the drug.

In fact, detoxing from drugs by quitting outright all of a sudden could even result in death. Detoxing from alcohol can be similarly dangerous, as it can cause symptoms of withdrawal that would feel similar to an illness and would almost certainly result in you being out of commission for a period of time.

Now it is time for you to understand the various symptoms that come with detoxing dangerously. Most of these symptoms come about as a result of detoxing too quickly due to the fact that you are consuming too many foods that aid in the detox process.

You might also be detoxing improperly, usually due to the fact that you are following an improper diet of some kind. Whatever the case may be, if you experience any of the following symptoms you will know that you are detoxing improperly in some way and should revert back to your normal diet.

Hair loss: Certain diets force you to leave certain nutrients out of your overall diet. These diets have been mentioned in this chapter before and should be avoided. A sign that you are not receiving enough nutrients is if you start to lose hair. This is a very extreme sign of malnutrition, and if you start experiencing abnormal hair loss during your detox diet stop detoxing immediately, revert to your original diet and preferably go see a doctor.

Skin irritation: This is another sign that you are running low on certain nutrients. Skin irritation is actually a normal part of detoxing, but if the irritation results in major breakage in your skin, in essence if the irritation is severe, then you are detoxing improperly and should stop immediately. However, if the skin irritation that you are facing is mild, for example a breakout of acne for a short period of time, then you have nothing whatsoever to worry about. Additionally, if you see red or pink patches on your skin during your detox period don't worry, as this is completely normal.

General irritability: You might start feeling cranky or irritable while you are on your detox diet. This is normal to a degree, as your body is craving the feel good chemicals that it was once able to get so easily and is now being deprived of. However, if your irritability turns into hostility, for example if you start experiencing violent mood swings, you will need to end your detox diet immediately. Improper detoxing can cause hormonal imbalances that can result in these sudden shifts in your mood.

Nausea or fever: A certain amount of nausea is to be expected while you are detoxing. Your body is getting rid of toxic chemicals that it has within it and this induces a feeling of nausea within you. However, vomiting is never supposed to happen while you are detoxing, and neither is fever. If either of these things happen to you while you are detoxing it means that your detox diet is improper and will result in a deterioration of your health. You are probably low on some kind of nutrient or are consuming too much detox food that is not agreeing with your body.

Weakness: While you are detoxing you can expect to feel a little lazy while the detox diet progresses. This is because your body has lost something that used to motivate it a lot. However, a detox diet is under no circumstances supposed to cause weakness in any form. If you begin feeling weak while you are on your detox diet, it probably means that you are not consuming enough calories which is resulting in your body being low on glucose and going into starvation mode. If you feel weak during your detox diet, try eating more while you are on it or stop in entirely.

Heart palpitations: Heart palpitations are a serious sign that something is wrong. They are not a normal part of detox diets in any way, and if you experience an irregular heartbeat you can rest assured that your detox diet is definitely not working out for you. Certain detox diets cause a deficiency in electrolytes that are necessary to keep the heart pumping efficiently and regularly. Go to a doctor and ask them if this was caused by a preexisting condition. If it wasn't, you need to change your diet immediately.

Depression: A little mood of depression is to be expected while you are detoxing because your body is so used to getting chemically induced shots of happiness hormones in its brain. It forgets how regulate the levels of serotonin and dopamine on its own, which means that for the first few days depression is normal. However, if it stretches on for more than four days, or if the depression gets extremely severe, you need to go see a doctor immediately. Ascertain the cause of the depression, and if it is being caused by your detox diet you will need to end it immediately.

Abdominal pain: There is absolutely no situation where abdominal pain is a normal part of a good detox diet. Abdominal pain is actually the opposite of what you should be feeling. Detox diets sometimes result in diarrhea, but this only lasts for a day or two at mist. If it lasts for longer, or if you start feeling any kind of abdominal pain, stop the diet immediately. You have probably become deficient in iron and fiber due to the nature of the particular diet that you are following, and continuing with the diet might end up causing irreparable damage to your digestive system.

Sore eyes: This is another sign that the diet that you are following is not quite right for you. Much like many of the other entries on this list, sore eyes are not, in fact, part of a normal detox diet. They are actually a sign that something dangerous is going on in your body caused by a deficiency in some nutrient or the other, more often than not this nutrient being vitamin C. If your eyes start becoming sore while you are on your detox diet, end the diet immediately, revert back to your original diet and go see a doctor immediately.

Constant drowsiness: As has been mentioned in a previous entry in this list, a little bit of laziness is a normal part of a detox diet as your body feels lethargic without the chemicals that made it feel so good. However, if you start feeling constantly drowsy you can be sure that the diet that you are is not good for you and that you should revert back to your original diet. Constant drowsiness can be the result of a hormonal imbalance or it can be the result of an unnecessarily low calorie intake. Either way, avoiding the diet that causes such a symptom is best.

Lowered immunity to disease: Another sign that your detox diet is absolutely not working for you is if you start getting sick a lot during the diet. Detox diets are never supposed to weaken your immune system, so if you start getting sick you can be sure that the diet you are following is not quite right. In general, if you can trace the origin of your sicknesses to the starting of your detox diet then you have definitely adopted a diet that is decidedly bad for you and should be changed if you don't want your health to deteriorate further.

Dizziness: Slight light headedness can be considered a normal part of the detox experience as your body is still getting used to functioning without all of those drugs and chemicals being poured into it. However, if you get so dizzy that you lose your balance you're in trouble. Detox diets are not supposed to have a profound effect on your balance, so unless you have a preexisting condition you should stop following your diet immediately and go see a doctor. Dizziness could be the result of a low consumption of calories, an extension of the aforementioned weakness, and should be taken seriously.

How Does Detoxing Help?

Now that you have come to learn about all of the dangers of detoxing, you are probably a little afraid to start detoxing yourself. After all, why would anyone attempt to do anything that could cause them so much harm?

The thing you need to realize is that all of the aforementioned dangers and negative symptoms are the result of improper detoxing, detoxing that involves unnecessary limitations on nutritional intake and forces you to abandon important parts of your diet. Such diets should be viewed as the opposite of what actual detoxing is supposed to do.

Yes, detoxing properly will actually have the complete opposite of all of the negative effects that have been mentioned in the previous chapter. In the worst case scenarios, you will get a taste of the milder negative symptoms, like skin irritation, and then your body will become accustomed to the chemical free way in which you are now living your life.

Hence, it is important to understand that detoxing is more about the good than the bad. All you need to do is to follow the proper ways in which you can detox, and you will be able to enjoy the following marvelous benefits:

> Better breath: Bad breath is one of the worst social faux pas that one can commit. It can put off dates, make people think less of you and just, in general, ruin your social life. This is probably even more frustrating for people when they realize that their bad breath is not even their fault! For some people, no matter how much they brush and how much mouthwash that they use, they simply can't get rid of their bad breath. This is actually because their colon is backed up. This is a little known cause of bad breath that actually has nothing to do with oral hygiene. Going on a detox diet clears out your colon if it is backed up, which will actually make your breath smell better once the diet is over. However, while the diet is ongoing remember that detox diets often cause bad breath. This is because the toxins are being expelled from your body and obviously are not going to smell very good! This is a normal part of the detoxing process, so just keep a breath mint or two handy and you'll be good to go.

> Alleviation of your chronic diseases: Chronic diseases are perhaps some of the most difficult things that people have to endure. They are lifelong companions, and rough ones at that, and living with them for a long time does tend to take its toll. Chronic illnesses can actually have a deep impact on your life, forcing you to adopt

different habits and in some ways can become a hindrance to your social life as well, especially if your chronic disease is particularly debilitating. However, if you detox properly you can actually reduce the symptoms of your chronic illnesses to the point where you will be able to live a completely normal life! Our chronic diseases may be caused by genetic anomalies but they are usually greatly exacerbated by the environment we surround ourselves in. The food we eat and the beverages we drink have a huge effect on the way our bodies handle these chronic illnesses. If you detox, you are freeing your body of toxins. These toxins that were clogging up your system force your body to handle them rather than your illness. Once they are flushed out, your body will be able to focus on its chronic problems instead, thereby making your symptoms a lot more bearable!

Enhancement of your immune system: This is partially tied to the previous amazing benefit that you receive from detoxing properly. Our immune system is what keeps us alive, it is an interconnected system of checks and balances that starts at our skin and is able to fight infections and diseases for a good long while, allowing us to live in the world without fear. However, our immune systems have recently started to become quite weak. This is mostly due to the creation of modern medicine. Modern medicine has slowly started to replace the work our immune system does with medicines which do the immune system's job for it. This is not to say that modern medicine doesn't save lives, it is an important part of why disease is so uncommon, only that we are becoming dependent on medicines. Detoxing allows you to boost your immune system by ridding your body of the substances that were getting in its way. The chemicals we consume make our already weakening immune system even more sluggish. By purging these chemicals, we allow our immune system to work at full capacity.

Weight loss: this may come as a surprise to you, particularly after previous chapters in which it is stated that weight loss is not what detox diets are for. This is actually true. The purpose of detox diets is never to lose weight, it is to purge your body of harmful chemicals. You should never start a detox diet with the intention of losing weight because that will warp the way that you approach the diet and might cause problems in the long run if you start to use detoxing incorrectly because you want it to make you lose weight. That being said, if you approach detoxing correctly and apply it with all of the correct rules and specifications, you will find that you will start to lose weight after a week or two of being on the diet. This is mostly because your metabolism gets stronger after the toxins have been flushed from your body, which means that your body can spend more time on metabolizing food without those toxins slowing it down. Additionally, the foods that you eat while you are on your detox diet are actually naturally not fatty or sugary, and thus allow you to lose weight while you are following this diet.

Slows down the aging process: We are living longer in today's modern day and age, thanks to modern medicine and its miracles, but at the same time we are aging quite quickly as well. This is simply due to the fact that the chemicals that we are consuming on a daily basis are simply toxic and are forcing our organs, especially our skin, to endure a lot more wear and tear than they would have otherwise. The things that we consume also contain a large amount of heavy metals as well as free radicals, both of which contribute heavily to the aging process. Detoxing, naturally, rids our bodies of these free radicals as well as these heavy metals that are polluting our systems, thereby allowing us to significantly slow down the aging process and prevent us from looking like we are forty when we are just thirty. This might just be a deal breaker for a lot of people considering the vain and vapid society that we currently live in which values physical beauty over anything else. Detoxing allows you to stay young while at the same time maintaining your youth in a natural and holistic way. It also doesn't hurt that detoxing can be considered a much, much cheaper alternative to all of these procedures that people go through in order to stay young.

Makes you feel better: We eat the things we eat and consume the things that we consume and throughout all of this consumption we do not realize that the joy that we are feeling is fleeting and temporary. The feeling of contentment we get after eating fast food is caused by the chemical makeup of that food, by the fact that the food has been specifically designed in order to make it stimulate the pleasure center of the brain. This is why we are never truly satisfied while we are living that lifestyle. We constantly crave another hit, no matter what it is that we are addicted to. Detoxing allows you to break that cycle. You feel true joy when your body is free of all chemicals and foreign toxins and is feeling the way it should feel. All of the joint pains and aches, all of the chronic diseases we develop, all of these go away when we detoxify our bodies because it is these toxins that were causing these problems in the first place!

Improves your energy: There are a large number of people out there whose number one complaint would be that they simply don't have enough energy throughout the day. They are unable to get up in the morning without drinking coffee, are unable to get through the day without some kind of stimulant that will help them gain enough energy to do the things that they need to do. This is mostly because of the toxins that have been built up inside them. These toxins prevent energy from being used efficiently by our bodies, which means that when you detox you are going to be discovering a whole fount of energy within you that you had never tapped before. Once the toxins are out of your body, your body will be able to process the foods that you are eating a lot more efficiently, it will be able to regulate your sleep patterns in a more efficient manner as well. You will find that you won't need to sleep as much, but while you do sleep it will be like a rock, and when you wake up you will be so fresh that you won't even need coffee or any of the other supplements that you had made a part of your morning kick start.

Improves your skin: This is an example of one of the negative things that could happen if you follow your detox diet improperly going absolutely right if you properly follow your detox diet with all of the rules and specifications that have been put in place in order to make it effective. If you follow a bad detox diet your skin will probably break out in acne and rashes and they simply won't go away until you stop following your diet. If you follow a proper detox diet, the result will actually be the same for the first couple of days. While your body is ridding itself of these toxins your skin might break in acne or rashes, but after they go away your skin will be positively glowing. All of the good things that you would have been putting into your system during your detox diet as well as all of the toxins that would be evacuating your body during this time would result in your skin clearing up, becoming naturally smooth and overall becoming the best skin without you having to resort to expensive beauty products.

Improved mental state: Eating all of these weird chemicals and substances definitely has an effect on your mental state. These chemicals alter the levels of chemicals in your brain, after all, so it can be assumed that your brain loses the ability to regulate itself. It becomes dependent on the fast food and drugs that you consume in order to boost its mood, and so it floods itself with depressant chemicals in order to balance your mental state out. However, since you cannot be eating fast food literally every second of the day, this probably gets you depressed and gives you a negative emotional and mental state. When you detoxify yourself, you will be depressed for a few days, but after this phase is ended you will feel absolutely fantastic, as though the world were at your feet. Your improved mental state will be the result of your brain being able to regulate its level of chemicals itself without the outside influence of the chemicals brought in by fast food, cigarettes or alcohol. Overall, detoxification allows you to feel like yourself again, and when it's over you will feel as though a fog has been lifted!

Chapter 12:

Other Ways to Detoxify

There is a misconception regarding what exactly detoxification is. Many people seem to think that detoxification involves following a strict diet where you are forbidden from eating certain kinds of food whereas other kinds of food you are strictly required to eat.

However the reality of the matter is actually much different. Detoxification does not quite require you to go on a diet. Rather it is more about avoiding the foods and drugs that make your body full of toxins and substances that slow it down and prevent it from doing the things it needs to do to keep you functioning.

Hence, it often comes as a surprise to people when they find out that there are several ways that they can detoxify their body without even having to alter their diets or change the way they eat in any significant way. In fact, these ways are often just as if not more effective than the detox diets that have become so popular as of late.

The main thing to remember with the following methods is that moderation is key. None of these methods are diets, and most of them require you to only change very minor details about your lifestyle.

Saunas

What a lot of people don't know about the detox process has a lot to do with the fact that they don't know much about how their body works. People think that toxins within their body are black swathes of sludge that cover their organs and arteries.

However, these toxins are actually not quite like that. They are actually trace chemicals that are in the blood stream, which means that they are a lot more insidious than a lot of people seem to understand because they are so difficult to pin point and tackle, which makes a lot of people think that altering the diet is the only way to go about expelling these substances.

However, there is another way to expel these toxins from your body, and that is through your sweat. When you sweat, your body removes all of the impurities that are just beneath your skin. Interestingly, this is where most of the toxins that we consume end up being deposited; just beneath our skin.

When we sweat, these impurities, the toxins that we are trying to get rid of, are expelled from our bodies without us even having to alter our diets in any way. Saunas are, therefore, one of the best ways to detoxify your body, particularly if you are looking for quick results. Try to go into the sauna for half an hour about three to five days per week.

Exercise

We are not a dumb species in general. We know what's good for us and what isn't, what we should do and what we shouldn't. We are more than aware of what we need to do in order to live long and healthy lives happily and without worry. Yet we do not pursue these options, we choose to fill our bodies with poison simply because they provide us with momentary pleasure.

This is probably why we usually avoid exercising. We know that it is good for us, we know that it can help make us a lot healthier, but we choose not to do it. However, it is important to note just how amazing exercise truly is.

Exercise is not just a way to lose weight quickly and in healthy amounts, it's not just a way to get healthier and stronger and to live a longer life. Exercise is one of the most effective ways to detox your body as well.

When we exercise, our body pumps blood and oxygen a lot faster because we need it. It is forced to work a lot more efficiently than it usually has to. This makes it efficient, but more importantly it also makes you sweat.

As you probably read under the previous subheading in this chapter, sweating really helps you to detox. Exercise is an even better way to sweat because the vigorously pumping blood is purified, allowing you to expel even more toxins than you would have been able to had you just sat there in the sauna.

Lemon water

As had been said just before this list of small things you can do to detox your body started, the most important things that we do in order to detox are often small. These involve tiny changes to the way we live our lives that help our bodies in enormous ways to flush the toxins out from within themselves.

One of these small things that you can do in order to help your body detoxify itself is to drink lemon water. Lemons are one of the most amazing fruits in existence. They contain copious amounts of vitamin C, and they are also chock full of antioxidants which, as you will probably remember from one of the previous chapters, is one of the best substances that you can have if you want to detoxify your body as they dissolve and weaken the toxic chemicals.

Vitamin C also increases a compound in the liver that greatly helps its job and helps to detoxify your body even further. It also doesn't hurt that water is possibly one of the most important detox drinks in the world because nothing else is quite as effective as water when it comes to diluting toxic chemicals and helping make the whole detoxification process easier for your body.

Try to drink all of your water with a bit of lemon in it. If not, try to have a couple of glasses of lemon infused water first thing in the morning and see just how well the rest of your day goes!

Avoid dairy

Dairy has always been considered the staple drink if you want to get healthy. Throughout our youths we were told that if we drank milk we would grow up to be big and strong, and to an extent it is true that milk helps us to become healthier. It is an important source of vitamin D and calcium and helps to make bones stronger. It is particularly important for children who are growing.

However, milk is also quite detrimental to the detoxification process. Drinking milk facilitates the buildup of mucus and it also makes the liver slow down its activities. The liver is one of the most important organs in the entire detoxification process, and so anything that makes it less able to do the important job that it does must be cut out.

Simply removing milk from your diet will help your body start to detoxify itself automatically. This may seem somewhat difficult, particularly considering that dairy products are such an important part of our ever day diets in this modern day and age, but if you really work at it you will find that it's actually not that difficult at all.

There are so many new options out there to traditional dairy products that you will soon find that you don't miss it at all. Soy milk as well as soy cheese are excellent alternatives to regular dairy products and don't clog up your liver at all!

Cut out the alcohol

We consume a lot of poisonous substances in our day to day lives. They make us feel good, help us to function in a lot of ways, and it is almost shocking how incredibly dependent we have become on these substances. It is particularly surprising considering that none of these substances are important for our survival, yet they are both more valuable and more sought after than food.

Perhaps none of these substances is as poisonous, nor as widely desired and celebrated, as alcohol. Alcohol is, plain and simple, a poison. The way it makes us feel when we consume it is a mild form of poisoning. However, we drink it as though we need it to survive, and in many ways we do because our social interactions, our confidence, all of these things seem to require alcohol.

Alcohol is one of the most severe sources of the toxins in our body out of all of the other substances that we consume, and cutting it out is possibly the best way to begin detoxing. After all, the first step to detoxing is actually stopping the consumption of poisonous toxins in the first place. When you stop consuming these toxins, your body will be able to start removing the toxins that are already present within it.

This also works if you quit smoking cigarettes. Stop filling your body up with the substances that harm it and you will find that it will start to heal itself automatically.

Cupping

This is perhaps one of the least known methods of detoxification these days, but that does not mean that it is the newest. In fact, cupping is one of the oldest methods of detoxification known to man, being practiced in the orient for over two millennia before the concept of detoxing became popular in the west.

The procedure is, for lack of a better word, somewhat radical, but it is also immensely effective. It can only be performed by a trained professional and must in no circumstances be tried at home because of the delicacy of the whole endeavor.

If you opt for the procedure, an expert will make a small cut in your back and place a small glass bowl with a flame inside it over the cut. The flame will burn up all of the air inside the bowl, creating a vacuum that would suck in blood from the cut.

This procedure may sound disgusting and painful but it is actually only the former of those things. It is not painful at all, and it is only disgusting because the blood that comes out will actually be quite dark and murky because it is dirty blood full of all of the toxins that you have consumed over the course of your life.

This is an extremely effective way to ensure that all of the toxins are pulled from your body, and it involves absolutely no changes to your diet whatsoever. However, the delicacy of the whole procedure just goes to show how dangerous the procedure can be if the proper precautions are not taken.

As long as you get cupping done by a trained professional, there is absolutely no harm and a great deal of good that it can do to you. Additionally, remember that everything is good in moderation. Too much cupping can definitely be bad for you because it can result in unnecessary blood loss.

Dry Brushing

This technique can actually go hand in hand with the very first technique mentioned in this list that involved sweating in a sauna in order to get rid of the impurities that have become piled up within our systems.

Dry brushing is basically what the name says it is. It involves taking a firm brush and very gently brushing your dry skin with it. This stimulates your pores and helps make them more efficient at what they do best: removing the impurities from within your body.

There are special brushes that come at herbal stores that are actually optimized to help you dry brush your skin and help your pores really open up and breathe, allowing you to relax while your body does the detoxing for you. This is a great example of how you can detox without having to resort to changing your entire lifestyle.

The reason that this can work so well hand in hand with the sauna technique is that sloughing off your dead skin in the sauna will help the steam reach your pores in an even more effective way. This means that the impurities will come out in even more copious amounts than they would have otherwise.

All of this is about improving the effectiveness of your body's own, natural detoxification process. Your body wants to be clean, and if you just give it the chance it will do all of the hard work for you!

Chapter 13:
Foods That Help in the Detox Process

There are certain foods that you can eat in order to make the whole process of detoxing easier and more efficient. Certain foods seem as though they have been created for the sole purpose of facilitating proper detoxification, and these foods are just what the doctor ordered if you feel as though your body is unable to function properly because of the fact that it is overflowing with toxins.

These foods are actually very easy to buy, and are virtually all fruits and vegetables. Here is a list of these foods in alphabetical order:

Artichokes: As you can probably tell by the amount of times it was mentioned in the previous chapter, the liver is pretty important as far as the whole process of detoxification goes, and artichokes are possible the best vegetables that you can eat in order to improve the functioning of your liver. At the very least, artichokes are one of the most important vegetables that help in this department. The way it helps the liver is that helps it to produce more bile, a substance that your body needs in order to successfully detoxify itself in an efficient manner.

Apples: As the saying goes, "An apple a day keeps the doctor away". There is a very good reason that this saying has come about, and that reason is that apples are just incredibly healthy fruits. Within their mealy flesh they have vitamins and minerals, not to mention fiber that not a lot of fruits have as well as a number of phytochemicals. These phytochemicals are incredibly important in the whole detoxification process, and are what make the apple such an important part of any detoxification diet. Just eat an apple in the morning and you'll be good to go!

Almond: Vegetables have been covered now as have been fruits, now all that is left is the nut category, and what an important category it is! Almonds are the kings of nuts because they are incredibly high in a specific form of vitamin E that helps boost the body's ability to detoxify itself. Additionally, almonds contain copious amounts of calcium and protein as well as the healthy and unsaturated variety of fatty acids. All in all, almonds are pretty much a super food and having a handful of almonds in the morning can help you detox as well as really improve your memory!

Asparagus: although being universally reviled by children everywhere, the asparagus actually doesn't taste all that bad. Asparagus is also, incidentally, an incredibly healthy food to eat because of the wide variety of benefits that it provides. It prevents cancer, first and foremost, but in this context the most important benefit that it provides is that it helps to drain your liver. Often when the toxins in our body are too high, the liver is unable to detoxify and gets backed up. Asparagus helps alleviate this issue by draining the liver!

Avocadoes: Avocadoes might just be one of the most delicious vegetables that money can buy. They also happen to be detox powerhouses, being packed with antioxidants and nutrients that don't just detoxify your body, lower your cholesterol and help clean up clogged blood vessels as well! One of the most important roles that avocadoes play is that they help the liver detoxify the body in a very specific way. A lot of fast food comes packed with synthetic chemicals, something avocadoes actually help the liver to break down. Hence, avocadoes play an especially important role in the struggle for a toxin free body!

Basil: Basil is not exactly a vegetable. In fact, it is more of a spice or an herb, and it is one of the most important herbs that you can possibly add to your food. One of the most important roles that basil plays is that it helps to protect the liver. The liver would obviously be unable to detoxify the body if it was sick, which means in protecting the sole organ that can help the body become a toxin free place, basil plays a role that is unspeakably important and very rarely ever credited.

Beets: If there was one vegetable in the entire vegetable kingdom that could be called a powerhouse, it would the beet. If the artichoke is the king of all vegetables, then the beet is the knight, powerful and multitalented. They are chock full of phytochemicals which help your liver remove toxins from within your body. Additionally, beets have the added benefit of purifying blood themselves, which means that they are able to help the liver do its job and help lessen its workload as well. Since the liver is possibly one of the most overworked organs in our bodies, beets are nothing short of a godsend.

Blueberries: No breakfast treat can be complete without the sprinkling of delicious blueberries on waffles or pancakes. What makes them so special is that they are actually natural painkillers, and they don't just deaden pain they lessen inflammation as well! The nutrients present within blueberries are extremely important for the liver, as they are special nutrients called phytonutrients that are specifically meant to nourish the liver and provide it energy while it detoxifies the body. The liver needs helpers, but it needs nutrients as well otherwise it won't be able to function!

Brazil nuts: often considered one of the tastiest nuts around, Brazil nuts are also packed with selenium. Selenium is mostly known for being able to flush out excess amounts of mercury from our system, but a little known other use that our bodies have for selenium is as a bit of a medic for our poor liver. While the liver does battle with the toxins, the selenium from Brazil needs patch up its wounds and helps it to recover from the strain of having to work so hard to clean up a body that is so chock full of toxins!

Broccoli: broccoli has been ingrained in the minds of children everywhere as being a yucky vegetable, and this time even us adults would tend to agree most of the time, unlike with asparagus that is actually fairly tasty. However, broccoli is actually an essential part of the entire process of detoxification because it specifically works by aiding the enzymes created by your liver to help flush the toxins from our bodies. These enzymes work by diluting the power of these toxins, breaking them apart and making them easier for the liver to manage. Detoxification wouldn't be possible without broccoli!

Brussels sprouts: Brussels sprouts are once again not quite the most delicious vegetables on the planet. However, what they do not possess in taste they make up for by being extremely important to the whole process of detoxification. Brussels sprouts contain certain phytochemicals that are also present in broccoli. However, Brussels sprouts contain these in much, much larger quantities. So where broccoli helps in creating the enzymes that break the toxins down, Brussels sprouts give the body, and the liver in particular, ammo to help fight the toxins when they appear in their weakened forms after going through the enzymes.

Cabbage: This may seem like a list of vegetables that you never want to eat, but rest assured that each of these vegetables is here for a reason. Cabbage is especially notorious for making people gassy, but it has a good reason for doing this. After all, it boosts the whole process of digestion and makes it a lot more efficient.

Not only does cabbage contain important chemicals that help the liver detoxify the body, they also help the body to excrete all of these toxins. After all, once the liver is done breaking the toxins down and weakening them, they have to be excreted otherwise there will have been no point.

Cilantro: this vegetable is also known as coriander, and is often used as more of a garnishing rather than an actual vegetable that people actively eat. One of the most important roles that cilantro plays is that it helps to get certain extremely dangerous toxins out of the body, toxins that the liver can't handle. These toxins are heavy metals such as mercury that are very poisonous for the body. Cilantro is also chocked full of antioxidants making it an excellent choice for your detox diet!

Cinnamon: one of the most fragrant and aromatic spices around, cinnamon is also famous, or rather infamous, for the cinnamon challenge in which people realized that cinnamon was, despite its sweet taste, a spice after all. It is also one of the foods with the richest concentration of antioxidants in the entire world. Incorporating cinnamon into your everyday life, such as drinking it in tea or sprinkling it over cake, is an excellent way to greatly boost your daily intake of antioxidants. Cinnamon also gives you a good energy boost, which is a nice bonus considering how much it detoxifies your body!

Cranberries: apart from inspiring the name of a famous Welsh pop band, cranberries have become famous for being old people fruits. This is because they greatly help in the prevention of urinary tract infections and help make the whole process of urination a lot easier. Additionally, in the context of detoxing, cranberries are extremely important because they provide very specific phytochemicals that few easily available fruits provide which greatly help the liver break down toxins and chemicals and process it into urine. Cranberries also help the body to excrete the toxins much in the same way cabbage does.

Dandelions: flowers in general are not considered food, and a flower as dainty and as delicate as a dandelion would certainly never be considered so. However, dandelions are extremely helpful for the liver in its struggle to break down toxins in order to make them easy to excrete. Their specific and rather unique nutritional makeup enables them to be extremely helpful to the liver because they help to strain the blood and rid it of toxins and wastes. This means that eating dandelion leaves with your salad would make it easier for your liver to do its job, and if any organ in our body deserves a break from time to time it's our liver.

Fennel: fennel is uniquely important to the liver's struggle against toxins as well, much in the same way dandelions are although its nutrients serve a different purpose. It provides a B vitamin called folate that helps to convert certain specific but extremely dangerous substances into benign molecules that the body can excrete without causing itself any major harm. Since fennel is such a concentrated source of folate as well as a specific anti microbial variant of vitamin C, it should make up a large part of your overall diet.

Flaxseeds: there has been a recent surge in the popularity of flaxseeds after their benefits were made known to the general public. One of their most important functions is that they provide wonderful, wholesome fiber that is essential to allowing your digestive system to excrete properly. As you already known, once the liver is done breaking the toxins down into more manageable and less dangerous or completely benign compounds, all that is left is that the body must excrete these toxins. Flaxseeds allow the body to do this in a more efficient manner.

Garlic: a favorite vegetable of both Italian as well as Indian cuisines! Despite being so far apart, these cuisines both seem to understand the importance of garlic, all of which lies in the fact that it helps boost the immune system while providing invaluable aid in the liver's struggle to break down toxins and make them benign enough to excrete. One of the most important elements of garlic is, perhaps, sulfur, which helps the liver create enzymes and provides invaluable support especially after you have a large amount of junk food and the liver is backed up in its attempts to clean up your system.

Ginger: Ginger is another staple of Indian cuisine although it is not equally celebrated in Italian cuisine the way garlic is. Possibly the most important role that ginger plays is that it helps the liver to get leaner. This is important when you consider the fact that we eat a lot more fat than we need. The liver tends to get a buildup of fat around it as a result. A fatty liver is unable to do its job properly, which means that if not for ginger our livers would be unable to detoxify our bodies at all!

Goji berries: these berries could potentially prove to be an alternative to raisins, a far healthier version at that. Goji berries possess a large amount of beta carotene that the liver really needs in order to do its job. Additionally, it aids the whole process of detoxification by providing the body with an enormous amount of vitamins. It is an extremely important source of vitamin C, which incidentally is one of the most important vitamins when it comes to flushing your body of toxins. A regular supply of goji berries can help you get healthier in no time!

Grapefruit: grapefruit possesses what can arguably be considered the most startlingly beautiful flesh of any fruit in world. However, it is equally bitter, even though the beauty of its flesh would imply sweetness. Much like many other entries in this list, the grapefruit makes up for the fact that it does not taste very good by being extremely good for you. It possesses a chemical called lycopene that is instrumental in the fighting of free radicals. This helps your liver get into its peak form within no time, making grapefruit an important part of every diet.

Green tea: As has been mentioned before, tea can be considered an important part of any detox diet because they contain so many anti oxidants. However, there is no tea in the world that has as many antioxidants as green tea. This is simply due to the fact that green tea is the least processed tea in the world. The leaves are almost exactly the way they were in the wild, all you do is boil them and drink the tea. The health benefits that green tea provides are massive, and the amount of help that the liver receives from it is similarly sized.

Hemp: Again, this food is yet another addition to the foods in this list that cannot be considered particularly tasty, however hemp is also one of the healthiest foods in the world. At least this time, the food does not taste bad, it's just tasteless! The most important role that hemp plays in the whole process of detoxification is that it keeps the digestive tract extremely clean. This allows the toxins to be broken down an excreted in an extremely efficient manner, something that would not have been the case had it not been for hemp.

Kale: once a complete unknown in the world of health, kale is now widely considered to be one of the most important foods in the world as far as detoxification is concerned. Kale has one of the highest concentrations of antioxidants in the world, and they are also chocked full of phytochemicals as well. The antioxidants help to purify the blood and the phytochemicals obviously help the liver to break down the toxins in the blood stream so that they do not cause any damage in the body's digestive system. Kale is truly a super food unlike any other!

Lemongrass: This herb is perhaps one of the oldest herbs that have ever been used for the purpose of cleansing the body. Used in the orient for at least hundreds of years, lemongrass has always been used for the specific purpose of cleansing organs of toxic chemicals. In fact, if you regularly consume lemongrass it will purge your entire digestive tract as well as your kidneys for you, meaning that your liver won't have to deal with any of this at all! Their cleaning of the digestive tract also makes it easier for the body to excrete toxic chemicals.

Lemons: Lemons are perhaps the poster boys of the entire detoxification movement, and for good reason too. They are instrumental for the liver to release its enzymes because the vitamins they contain are just so good for the liver. Lemons also induce the creation of alkaline chemicals in our digestive system, which is very important especially after we have eaten particularly spicy or rich foods that will be causing a lot of acidity. In general, lemons are perhaps the most important fruits that we can eat in our quest to detoxify our body and free ourselves of all foreign chemicals.

Olive oil: India got two, now Italy gets its second celebrated food in olive oil. It is one of the healthiest oils that you can use and is actually quite good at helping the liver to do its job and detoxify the body. It is low in fat and actually triggers a detoxification response in the liver, which is very important particularly when you are starting a detox diet. Even eating olive oil with your pizza or cooking your pasta in it can do your health a world of good, as olive oil is the healthiest oil that you can use.

Onions: Here we have a vegetable that is a stable for cuisines from around the world, and there is good reason for that. Not only are onions deliciously sharp, they are extremely healthy as well. The particular type of amino acids that onions contain provides a very specific benefit to the liver, which is that it detoxifies it. That's right, with all that detoxification the liver actually gets pretty toxic too! The onion helps it to become healthy and helps it to do its job as well, adding yet another vegetable into the category of super food.

Parsley: This is another example of a vegetable that is generally used as garnishing instead of being eaten outright that actually deserves to be eaten due to the immense health benefits that it provides. Chock full of vitamins A, B and even K, as well as large amounts of beta carotene, parsley is perhaps one of the most important vegetables you can eat while you are attempting to detox. Parsley also helps the body to reduce the amount of free radicals it has within it as well that helps to improve overall health and make the detoxification process a lot easier.

Pineapples: A delicious entry into this list at last! Pineapples aren't just one of the tastiest fruits around, they contain a little thing called bromelain which is absolutely essential to the health of your body and the detoxification process in general. Bromelain is a digestive enzyme that, of course, helps your body digest food. This means that it helps to cleanse the colon as well as the entire digestive tract that is an extremely important part of the detoxification process because it allows the body to flush the toxins that it has within it more efficiently.

Seaweed: Seaweed has recently come to be known as somewhat of a super food as well, with a lot of health experts beginning to promote it as being a great vegetable to eat. Indeed, it has been one of the most underrated vegetables for the longest time, especially considering the fact that it is able to bind itself to radioactive materials within our bodies and excrete them safely. This unique power of seaweed makes it an absolute must eat for us especially considering that we have absolutely no idea what it is that we are actually eating these days!

Sesame seeds: They are part of every good bun and add a savory goodness to them that we have come to take for granted, but sesame seeds are also extremely important because they are chock full of enzymes and antioxidants as well as important minerals, all of which are absolutely essential in our livers' struggle to dilute and break down the toxins that are present in our body. Sesame seeds also contain anti inflammatory agents which are very useful if you are suffering from swelling in any area of your body and don't want to use medicine.

Turmeric: this spice is essential because it aid both the liver as well as the digestive system. Its unique blend of nutrients is useful because it helps to optimize the liver's potential, allowing it to function at its maximum capacity. It also cleans out your digestive system, allowing your body to excrete the toxins it has within it in a more efficient manner. This double team of clean digestive system and optimum liver functionality is further boosted by the high antioxidant count that turmeric possesses. What all of this means is that turmeric should really be in your food!

Watercress: This vegetable is extremely important for your liver because it helps it to release the enzymes that it possesses within it and break down the toxic chemicals that have been built up within your body. It also possesses a lot of antioxidants that further help your body to detoxify itself.

Wheatgrass: This food is really important because of how much alkalinity it brings to your entire system. It works by reducing the acidity in your overall blood that is a very important way in which your body can detoxify itself, as toxins within your blood can make your blood acidic.

Chapter 14:

How Not to Detoxify Your Body –
10 Ways

While drinking water is a good detoxification measure, by itself it is not enough to get rid of the toxins you take n on a daily basis. There are plenty of other things that you need to be doing but there are also some things that you should be aware of. Going gung-ho into a detox plan will not work if you don't plan for it. Take not of these 10 ways on how NOT to detoxify your body.

1. Go Extreme

During a detox, you are going to be changing the way you eat, drink and behave but you do not need to go to extremes to accomplish this. Many people believe that a detox requires them to star themselves for a period of time and that it's going to hurt. This is not the case. The most successful detox plan will have you focusing on being calm and feeling well and healthy while feeding your body the nutrients it requires. Starving yourself will NOT achieve that.

2. Be Unprepared

Having the wrong attitude when it comes to detoxing your body is the fastest path to failure because you simply won't get the results you want. You must be prepared and you must know exactly what your plan is. Ask yourself these questions:

- How am I going to achieve this?

- How am I going to start?

- How long will I do this for?

- How will I get back to normal afterwards?

Of course, "normal" is going to be different so you need to work out what your new "normal" is going to be, Will you go back to how you were before or will you use this chance to change your ways? Ask yourself all of these questions and more before you start or you simply will not succeed.

3. Pick the wrong time to start

It is no good planning to start a detox plan when you are stressed out or at a busy time in your life. If you have a birthday coming up or the holidays are approaching, don't start a detox, wait until afterwards. Pick a time when there are likely to be few temptations and no distractions otherwise you simply will not stick to it and you will not reap any of the benefits. After holidays, after big parties or when you can take time off work and chill out are the best times.

4. Forget the water

It really doesn't matter which plan you choose to go with when you detox, there is one thing that is included in all of them – water. You may have to drink more water than you usually do but you must make the conscious effort to do so. Water is vital at any time but even more so when you are detoxing. This is because your organs are detoxing and need to get rid of the unhealthy impurities and toxins they are loaded with. They cannot do this if they do not have sufficient water to keep them hydrated. Drinking water regularly throughout the day helps to keep your internal workings running smoothly and to make sure you get enough water at a time when you may have to reduce your intake of food.

5. Ignoring the signals your body is sending

While you should always take note of your body, when you detox it is especially important. If, during your plan, you start to feel uncomfortable or in pain that is more than just hunger, do not continue pushing on and try to get past the pain. Speak to your doctor before you start a detox plan, as it may not be suitable for you or there may be contraindications that you need to be aware of. That way, you will be more certain about the pain, whether it is because of the detox or something else. You do need to be healthy to do a detox and if anything doesn't seem right, stop and, if necessary, seek medical advice

6. Rush in and rush out of a detox program

Both your mind and your body have to be ready for a detox so never rush in and just suddenly stop eating, or start of fruits and vegetables only for days and days on end. Your body needs to be eased in, to give it a chance to understand that things are changing. You must also prepare your mind for the changes ahead so it does not send your body into panic mode. At the other end of the plan, do not just rush out and go back to a normal diet. Again, you must ease your body back into it otherwise it will go into shock, especially if you start eating foods that you haven't eaten for several days.

7. Forget about your mind

So many people think that detoxing is just about the body and they forget about their minds. You can detox you mind just as well as you can your body. It's all about banishing negative thoughts, harmful thoughts and upsetting information and increasing the flow of positive information. Try doing a detox while watching the news when it's full of bad news and you will find that you will not be anywhere near as successful as you should be. You must detach yourself from all negative influences and relax.

8. Give in to the cravings

When you detox you are stopping the harmful flow of toxins into your body so it will do you no good whatsoever if, just after you start or halfway through, you give in to the inevitable cravings that will hit. It is only natural for your body to crave what you have always given it, especially when you suddenly take that substance away without warning. A good program will acknowledge your cravings and it will have a system for you to follow when those cravings hot. It will be a soup, a smoothie or a tea that can take the place of the food you crave.

Look at it this way – cravings are an excellent sign that the detox is working. Fight back against your body's screams and you will emerge triumphant and keep in mind that cravings only last a few minutes.

9. Keep switching between detox programs

You might think that the program you are eon is not working or that another plan looks far better, especially when you are halfway through it. What you must do, before you start on another plan, is finish the one you are on. You might not need to do another one if you let your current one run its course properly. Stopping and starting all the time will not get you the results you desire and you will not be any healthier.

Follow a program from start to finish and then leave it a while to assess the results before you jump straight in to another one. Giving up one plan for another is generally seen as a type of escape mechanism, one that allows you to get out of a program when the going gets a little too tough for you and you are unlikely to ever successfully complete a program.

10. Give it all up too soon

While it is important that you do not ignore the signals that your body is sending out, it is also important that you do not throw the towel in and give it all up when things start to get a little rough. More often than not, it is when you have got through a rough stage that the real detoxing and cleansing begins and you start to see the real positive effects of what you are doing. You must be able to work out what is considered normal and what isn't when it comes to the side effects of detoxing. Really and truthfully, to understand that, you need to be there throughout the entire process and that is the only way you are going to get the results that you are looking for. If necessary, join a couple of forums and get advice, support and help from those that have been there and successfully completed it.

These are the 10 biggest mistakes that are made by people starting out on a new detox program, especially in those that have never done one before. Avoiding these mistakes will make it more likely that you will succeed and you will reap the benefits from your detox program. Do not underestimate the ability that your body has in recovering from whatever you throw at it. The human body is remarkably resilient and stronger than you give it credit for. Al you are doing is giving it a helping hand, a respite from the hard work it does for you and it will respond positively when it knows that you are looking out for it. Keep that positive thought in your mind and success will be yours.

Conclusion

O nce again, thank you for downloading my book. I hope that I have been able to give you an oversight of what a detox is, how it works, and why we need to do it on a regular basis.

Anyone who is looking to kick start their weight loss, cleanse their systems so they feel better or simply give them back their youthful appearance will benefit from a detox cleanse. I must just reiterate that you should never carry out these plans long-term unless it is specified that you can. A proper diet detox can be done long term but those of you who are choosing the fruit or water detox must not go any further than 3-5 days without eating some form of proper food.

Please remember to seek medical advice if you are all unsure about whether a detox is right for you or if you have any condition that could make it dangerous. Your health is the most important thing and, although this is why we do a detox, doing one can worsen certain conditions.

CPSIA information can be obtained
at www.ICGtesting.com
Printed in the USA
BVHW091049180321
602887BV00010B/1220